EAT TO FOCUS

The Not-so-Obvious Natural ADHD Treatment Protocol to Reduce Hyperactivity & Impulsivity, and Better Focus and Memory Without Drug Side Effects

by

Anna O. Tai, RD, CD, CSP.

Copyright © 2021 by Anna O. Tai

All rights reserved. This book or any portion thereof
may not be reproduced or used in any manner whatsoever
without the express written permission of the publisher
except for the use of brief quotations in a book review.

Perfect Homes Honolulu LLC, 2021

ISBN: 9798629655299

TABLE OF CONTENT

INTRODUCTION 6
Why am I Writing This Book?

WHAT DOES ADHD IN CHILDREN LOOK LIKE? 20
Is It ADHD or Something Else?
Why is My ADHD Child Always Hungry?
The Scary Truth About Untreated ADHD

CONVENTIONAL ADHD TREATMENT 45
How Does ADHD Medication Work?
Is ADHD Medication Safe?

FUNCTIONAL ADHD TREATMENT 54
6 Possible Root Causes of ADHD
Every Child Is Different
Nutrition Comes First

EAT TO FOCUS PROTOCOL 151
Why Follow the Eat to Focus Protocol

PHASE 1 - CLEAN START 166
Minimize Environmental Toxins
Remove Trouble Food

PHASE 2 - FEED THE ADHD BRAIN 200
Eat Real Food
Stabilize Blood Sugar
Correct Nutrient Deficiencies

PHASE 3 - FEED THE ADHD GUT 254
Patch Up Leaky Gut
Correct Poor Digestion
Correct Gut Bacteria

PHASE 4 - BRAIN REBOOT 267
Brain Gym
Quiet Time Quiet Mind
Healing Hours

EAT TO FOCUS QUICK START GUIDE 308

ADDITIONAL RESOURCES 328

APPENDIX 331
Food Intake & Symptom Tracker
Brain Kryptonite Foods to Avoid
Rocket Fuel for the ADHD Brain
ADHD-Friendly & Kid-Friendly Snack Ideas

BONUS CHAPTERS 355
How to Get Your Picky Eater to Eat Anything
Brain Boosters to Maximize Brain Power

SCIENTIFIC REFERENCES 409

This book is dedicated to all the great parents who are brave enough to take on this divine role of bringing up a human being or two and helping him or her to be the best he or she can be through your sacrifices and dedications.

No one can understand the feeling of being a parent until you became one. They say a child is a gift from God. A child changes your whole world and makes you a better person.

Thank you for being great parents!

The world is better because of you and your children.

INTRODUCTION

Hey there!

I'm so excited that you are here.

My name is Anna Tai. I'm a Registered Dietitian and Board-certified Specialist in Pediatric Nutrition. I'm also a parent of a child with ADHD like you.

MY STORY

I was in your shoe many years ago…desperate and frustrated.

I know something was not right, but I don't want to get her tested and diagnosed. Somewhere deep down inside me I know there are better options, and medication is not one of them.

Since the beginning, I figured she is different.

My daughter was super active since she's started moving. She started walking around seven months and was climbing up and down everything. She never sits still. The only time she is not moving is when she's sick. She'd dash out into traffic or runoff in stores and airports. It scared the crap out of me. One second you saw her, next second she's gone.

I'm those people who think parents who put their kid on a leash are loser parents, and I wouldn't do that to my child.

Man, am I wrong?

My daughter was out of control when she was a toddler. She's always on the go, climbing up and down every piece of furniture, pulling things off of shelves and tables, and breaking everything in the house.

Every morning was an ordeal. I, a grown woman, and her dad, a grown man, could not get her out of her pajama. We would have to drop her off at the daycare in her pajama with her change of clothes, so the nice "aunties" at the daycare could change her later.

And I felt so sorry for the lovely ladies at the daycare every day dealing with her. My daughter would cry from the moment we leave the house on the 20 minutes car ride until we arrive at the daycare.

The ladies at the daycare were so sweet and always reassured me that "don't worry, she usually cried for about 20 minutes, then she'd stop."

Bless her heart.

The crying started again when I picked her up from daycare because she realized it was so much fun there, she did not want to leave.

So again, crying all the way home.

Then, there's the non-stop crazy crying and screaming. I didn't know what my daughter wants. She would scream and cry for whatever reason I had no idea.
She also didn't start talking until almost two years old, and her first word is "apple." I wish I'd know to teach her sign language back then, so she could communicate better. She was in speech therapy for a few years, mostly for speech delay. She was also behind in reading and writing compared to her peers.

The ADHD symptoms become more obvious in elementary school. She took a long time to finish homework. We stayed up late until midnight every night. I have PTSD when I hear the word "homework." She could not read at, and she could barely write at her grade level. I feel so frustrated because I was comparing her to her peers.

Why can't you just finish the sentence? Why can't you pronounce the word?

We enrolled her in every reading and writing program during school breaks. I signed her up for piano lessons hoping that the music will help calm her down and sitting still. She was an outstanding and quick learner. But she didn't have the patience to practice. She played the piano like it's a typing speed contest.

She also started playing tennis to let out energy at the end of the day. She's an excellent tennis player but made many simple mistakes because of her lack of focus.

Then, I started working in the Feeding Clinic alongside the speech pathologist and other pediatric developmental specialists. That's when I learned that children who cannot focus usually have speech and language delay because they cannot sustain their focus long enough to pay attention to learn the words or sentences.

I also started to specialize in children's nutrition and started seeing many kids with special needs, such as inborn error of metabolism, genetic disorders, autism, ADHD, oral aversion, etc.

Most of the kids with ADHD I see are for failure to thrive (problem growing and not growing weight). I started to notice one particular psychiatrist was doing something very different than other doctors and psychiatrists.

He was prescribing coffee and this new prescription fish oil. This fish oil was marketed for heart disease prevention in adults.

So I started looking into coffee and fish oil for ADHD. What I discovered blew my mind.

That's when I realized "coffee is a stimulant just like ADHD medications, so why are we giving kids such dangerous stimulant drugs instead?"

That was my "aha" moment.

TO MEDICATE OR NOT MEDICATE?

When you have high blood pressure or pre-diabetes, your doctor often gives you a warning and likely suggests that you start eating healthier and exercising.

Why don't they do the same for kids with ADHD?

Did you get a warning first to change your child's eating and lifestyle?

Why is every doctor so quick to start ADHD medication, which has more severe side effects?

If parents are concern about giving children coffee because "coffee supposedly causes stunt growth", you should be even more concerned about giving children ADHD medications.

ADHD medications not only cause stunt growth, but also cause sleep disorder, mood disorder, personality changes, facial tics, etc…and, even death.

In March of 2006, an FDA panel reported that 11 sudden cardiac deaths in children taking Ritalin and Concerta between 1992 and 2005. Both medications contain the stimulant methylphenidate. They also reported 13 sudden cardiac deaths among children taking the amphetamine-containing stimulants Adderall and Dexedrine.

Coffee is a natural stimulant.

ADHD medication is a synthetic (man-made) stimulant in the same drug category as amphetamine (street drug "ice"). Just because a doctor prescribes it does not make it safer or better.

I started doing my research and experimenting with my poor child, and I discovered many possible causes of ADHD, which can easily be corrected with dietary changes and lifestyle changes.

And you know what?

It worked for us.

My daughter graduated from one of Hawaii's most prestigious private school with honors. Her public school teacher told us that she would not make the cut to be accepted to this school. It's a very competitive and selective school.

Not only did she graduated with honors, but she also received a hefty merit scholarship to attend Loyola Chicago University. She's currently a junior majoring in pre-med, with plans to continue onto medical school to become a pediatric cardiologist.

I am not bragging here. *I just want to share my experience with you, so you know there is hope and what is possible for your child too.*

Our result was not pure luck. It was a long journey of trial-and-errors, believing and not giving up.

These is no magic potion. And you don't need to be a Ph.D. to figure out what to do. You just need the right strategy.

Your child deserves the best, and you can help.

Stay strong and keep believing your child. He or she is doing their best. Your child just needs one person to believe in them, and that's you.

I've helped hundreds of my own ADHD patients improve their symptoms with my signature *Eat to Focus Protocol*, which you'll learn in this book.

Having the right strategies is like having *Neiman Marcus Chocolate Chip Recipes*. You don't need to go to a fancy French pastry school for years to figure out how to make the best cookies in the world.

It breaks my heart to see children suffer. Parents worry about caffeine stunt growth. I've never in my 18 years professional career know a child with stunt growth because of caffeine.

But I can look at the growth chart of any child with ADHD and tell you exactly when the child started ADHD medications.

Caffeine is used as a lung surfactant in brand new premature babies in the neonatal intensive care unit (NICU) every day. So giving children caffeine is not a new or unusual practice. It's a common practice in all NICUs everywhere.

So why can't we try some caffeine or other natural stimulant first before ADHD medications?

Unlike the common belief that coffee makes you hyper, it does the opposite for kids and adults with ADHD. Caffeine helps them to calm down and focus.

If you're a coffee drinker yourself, you know what I'm talking about.

I just want to be clear here. I'm not advocating coffee as "THE ALTERNATIVE" ADHD treatment. Besides, you build up a tolerance to coffee quickly.

Coffee or caffeine is just a quick fix for ADHD symptoms and could be an alternative to synthetic stimulants.

One of the doctors in my clinic drinks 10 cups of coffee a day. No kidding…he told me himself. He has a Keurig next to him on his desk.

One of my previous supervisors drinks 2 liters of diet Mountain Dew a day.

Yes, I counted it every day.

There are better ways to get your child to calm down and focus naturally without ADHD medications.

If there are no other options, and ADHD medications are the only choice. That's a different story.

CONVENTIONAL VS FUNCTIONAL APPROACH

Have you ever tried a supplement that you read about in Facebook groups and recommendations from friends, who swear that such supplements work for their children, but do nothing for them?

Does the supplement improve your child's ADHD symptoms a little, but not the explosive and aggressive behaviors?

Most people's idea of alternative approaches to treating ADHD symptoms is limited to behavioral interventions, neurofeedback, taking some fish oil, magnesium, and some multivitamins. They merely replace the dangerous ADHD meds with a perceived "less dangerous" herbal natural alternative and call it natural ADHD treatment.

There's more to natural ADHD treatment than just popping some vitamin pills and going to therapy. I'm not saying these do not work ...it's just may not work for your child.

The *Eat to Focus Protocol* focuses on identifying and correcting the underlying causes of ADHD of the individual child.

Even though everyone gets diagnosed with ADHD are diagnosed based on the same set of observed symptoms, not everyone has the same underlying causes.

That's why even the current conventional treatment does not work for everyone either.

ADHD medications work by hijacking your child's control center (the big brain in the head), which explains why the typical personality change "not feeling like myself" seen in kids taking ADHD meds.

If you feel like you're randomly throwing spaghetti at the wall and see what sticks, the conventional treatment is just about the same by targeting the neurotransmitters in the brain and see if it works for your child.

Conventional medicine focuses on treating the symptoms of ADHD. Here, we're going to teach you to use clues (signs) to identify your child's underlying causes.

If you're just focusing on finding the next "natural pill of the day" for your ADHD treatment, you're missing a massive piece of the ADHD puzzle.

We all know the ADHD brain is different, but did you know there's also an ADHD gut?

ADHD IS NOT JUST IN THE BRAIN

Scientists are now learning more about the gut-brain axis and have established that our gut is possibly our second brain, and is as essential as the first brain on our shoulder.

Many kids with ADHD do well with the standard ADHD supplements for the usual ADHD symptoms, such as lack of focus, poor memory, fidgeting, etc.

However, the more explosive and aggressive ADHD symptoms, such as anger outbursts, impulsivity, aggressiveness, agitation, anxiety, and emotional meltdowns, seem to originate from the ADHD gut, which requires drastic dietary changes to correct.

If ADHD medication makes your child's ADHD symptoms worse, chances are the causes are in the gut.

Taking nutritional or dietary supplements without making dietary changes is like eating poison while also taking antidotes daily.

It's just a matter of time that the body stops responding to the antidote.

If what you've just read makes sense to you, keep reading. The best has yet to come.

Even though every doctor starts anyone with "ADHD" with the same stimulant no matter what their ADHD symptoms are, they are hyperactive or inattentive or whatever.

All children with ADHD get the same treatment because they all have the same diagnosis (or label), right? That's our medical system right now.

In my book, there is no "one size fits all," then there's certainly no "one diet fix all" either.

I'm used to looking at an individual's unique biology and symptoms to see the best treatment to start.

I applaud you for choosing the arduous journey to help and support your children in the most natural ways.

Natural ADHD treatment is not just about finding the right diet or the right supplements for your child.

It's not about getting your child to sit still through a boring class to please the school or the teacher.

It's about doing what is best for your child. This journey is all about your child's future.

I'm not against ADHD medication. Some children need it. But there are better alternatives for others.

I hope with this book, I can empower you with information to make the best treatment choices for your child by better understanding the underlying causes and natural treatment options available.

A lot of heartache and lives can be saved just by being an informed medical consumer.

Knowledge is power.

Aloha with love,

Anna

WHAT DOES ADHD IN CHILDREN LOOK LIKE?

My head was hurting at the end of the session. This particular boy was here for his weight, but the whole time he was *bouncing in the chair, legs fidgeting, interrupting my conversation* with his mom, and *non-stop talking* about some topics of interest to him at the moment.

Does this sound familiar? Keep reading.

ADHD stands for *Attention Deficit Hyperactivity Disorder.* It is a neurological and mental disorder associated with *the inability to focus or concentration on regular daily tasks*.

ADHD or ADD is usually diagnosed in childhood. We all know young children have a short attention span. But if his/her attention span is unusually short-spanned for his/her age, that warrants some concern. Or an older child who cannot stay put in his/her chair, and he/she behaves more like a toddler wandering around the classroom.

A diagnosis of Attention Deficit Disorder (ADD) means your child has a hard time focusing WITHOUT being hyperactive. But, in general, ADHD and ADD are used interchangeably.

ADHD in children can affect learning, self-esteem, and social skills. It is essential to get proper diagnosis and treatment early.

Diagnosis of ADHD is usually based on behaviors observed by parents, teachers, and care providers. And the child is generally evaluated by an experienced child psychiatrist.

Do you know someone who is forgetful, gets distracted easily, talks a lot and very fast?

We all know someone who we think has ADHD because of certain behaviors.

I once had a coworker who talks very fast. When I first met him, I couldn't understand what he was saying. I drew a total blank trying to figure out what language he was speaking because I could not understand a word coming out of his mouth. He literally talked like Twitchy in *Hoodwinked*.

And one time, my boss asked me to give him a ride to the car dealership to pick up his car. I swear to God, I barely uttered a syllable during the whole 30 minutes car ride. He talked non-stop at 1,000 miles per hour about something, which I probably didn't care about.

Does my coworker or boss have ADHD?

According to the DSM-5 criteria for ADHD diagnosis, the *inattention and/or hyperactivity and impulsivity* symptoms have to be persistent and *interfere with children's daily functioning or development*.

To be considered **inattentive**, you have to have at least six or more symptoms of inattention for children up to age 16, or five or more for adolescents 17 and older and adults for at least six months. These symptoms have to interfere with your life or inappropriate for your age:

- *Often fails to give close attention to details or makes careless mistakes in schoolwork, at work, or with other activities.*

- *Often has trouble holding attention on tasks or play activities.*

- *Often does not listen when spoken to.*

- *Often does not follow through on instructions and fails to finish schoolwork, chores, or duties in the workplace (e.g., loses focus, side-tracked).*

- *Often has trouble organizing tasks and activities.*

- *Often, it avoids, dislikes, or is reluctant to do tasks that require mental effort over a long time (such as schoolwork or homework).*

- *Often loses things necessary for tasks and activities (e.g., school materials, pencils, books, tools, wallets, keys, paperwork, eyeglasses, mobile telephones).*

- *Get distracted easily*

- *being forgetful in daily activities.*

For a child under 16 years of age, you have to have at least six or more hyperactivity/impulsivity symptoms.

For adolescents 17 and older and adults, you have to have at least five or more symptoms for at least six months, and these symptoms have to interfere with your life or inappropriate for your age:

- *Often fidgets with or taps hands or feet or squirms in seat.*

- *Usually leaves place in situations when remaining seated is expected.*

- *Often runs about or climbs in situations where it is not appropriate (adolescents or adults may be limited to feeling restless).*

- *Often unable to play or take part in leisure activities quietly.*

- *often "on the go" acting as if "driven by a motor."*
- *Often talks excessively.*

- *Often blurts out an answer before the question was finished.*

- *Usually has trouble waiting his/her turn.*

- *Often interrupts or intrudes on others (e.g., butts into conversations or games)*

How many of the above symptoms of ADHD does your child have?

Wait...this is meant for educational purpose only, not for you to self-diagnose.

Besides, there are still other criteria to meet and evaluations by a trained psychiatrist.

So if you have a few of the above symptoms of ADHD and these symptoms have persisted for six months or more, and they're affecting your social life, work function, or school, talk to your primary care physician for a proper diagnosis.

We all can find a few of these behaviors in ourselves at some point in time, such as *not getting enough sleep* will cause you to make more mistakes during the day, *life stresses* can also result in more inattentive behaviors, etc.

To understand ADHD more, think of the brain as having crisscrossing wires that go in many directions. For most people, a thought moves directly from point A to point B.

For someone with ADHD, a thought starts at point A, but before it gets to point B, it may have stopped at multiple pit stops at points C, point D, and maybe even point E. They become entirely distracted before point B.

That sounds like me. I often make multiple stops before getting to the kitchen where I want to go.

Can you relate?

This so-called "wiring defect" creates two common problems seen in children with ADHD:

1. Poor executive function

Projects with many steps are often overwhelming for a child with ADHD, who doesn't know where to start. They end up procrastinating or never even start or started a project and never finished.

2. Poor self-regulation

A child with poor self-regulation lacks impulse control and might do things without first considering consequences. They act on a random thought impulsively.

Most people think that ADHD is a lack of attention, which is often the misconception of ADHD. But a child with ADHD can pay attention. The problem is that a child with ADHD is interested in nearly everything they hear and see. Sometimes they are so focused on one fascinating subject that they block out everything else and "hyperfocus" on that one thing.

To parents and teachers, this looks like a child with ADHD is day-dreaming, ignoring them, and not listening.

There are also other symptoms commonly seen in children with ADHD that are not necessarily included for the diagnosis.

These other symptoms include anger, agitation, anxiety, aggressiveness, mood swings, depression, etc.

Is It ADHD or Something Else?

Did you know more than two-thirds of individuals with ADHD have at least one other coexisting condition?

In fact, "pure ADHD" cases are relatively uncommon.

As part of diagnosing ADHD, your child's doctor should also be assessed for other conditions based on your child's symptoms.

Growing up, my daughter had quite a few incidences in schools, and one of the scariest moments was when I received a phone call from my daughter's teacher one afternoon. She threatened to call the police to arrest my daughter because she bit one of the students and left a bite mark on her arm.

She was only 6-7 years old at the time. They're just fooling around according to the girls. This teacher already called the other student's parent, who did not want to push charges.

My daughter tends to be a little wilder and rougher than other kids when it comes to playing.

I worked with children with special medical needs, so I see children with all kinds of medical and developmental disorders daily. I definitely can identify a few traits of the mental disorders in my child.

Do you see your child in any of these conditions?

The symptoms of ADHD, such as constant movement and fidgeting, interrupting and blurting out, difficulty sitting still, etc., may overshadow these other coexisting conditions.

Just as untreated ADHD can be challenging in everyday life, these other coexisting conditions can also cause unnecessary suffering in individuals with ADHD and their families.

Any conditions can coexist with ADHD, but certain conditions tend to happen more frequently with ADHD. And ADHD does not cause other psychological or developmental conditions. They happen together likely because they have similar root causes.

Many times, symptoms of ADHD can masquerade as other diagnoses.

For example, people with ADHD often have "mood swings" and difficulty with mood regulation, which isn't included in the DSM IV criteria.

When someone with ADHD is sad or in a funk, they have a hard time shaking it. And when they are excited, they are really excited.

This is one of the gifts and wonderful traits of people with ADHD. They are passionate people, passionate about life and passionate about letting other people know about it.

If you don't know this person well, you might think this person has bipolar disorder, which is very common in people with ADHD.

However, more often than not, people with ADHD who say they have mood swings, just mean "ADHD mood swings" not the bipolar manic swings.

1. Learning Disabilities

Up to 50 percent of children with ADHD have a co-existing learning disorder compared to only 5 percent of children without ADHD. Learning disorders can cause problems with how individuals acquire or use new information such as reading, writing, or calculating.

The most common learning disorders in children with ADHD are dyslexia and dyscalculia. About 12 percent of children with ADHD may also have speech problems, compared to only 3 percent of children without ADHD.

Diagnosing learning disabilities requires specific academic testing, which is usually done by a psychologist.

2. Oppositional Defiant Disorder (ODD)

As many as 30% to 50% of all children with ADHD have oppositional defiant disorder (ODD). These children are often disobedient, rebellious, and hostile toward authority figures and have random outbursts of temper.

ODD involves a pattern of arguing, losing one's temper, refusing to follow the rules, blaming others, deliberately annoying others, and being angry, resentful, spiteful, and vindictive. Also, ODD is more common in boys than girls.

3. Conduct Disorder

Conduct disorder is a more severe form of antisocial behavior. Approximately 27 percent of children, 45-50 percent of adolescents, and 20-25 percent of adults with ADHD have conduct disorder (CD).

Children with conduct disorders frequently lie or steal, tend to disregard others' welfare, and risk getting into trouble. Children with conduct disorder may be aggressive to people or animals, destroy property, run away, or skip school and destroy properties.

4. **Anxiety Disorders**

Anxiety disorders are associated with an overwhelming sense of worry and nervousness and obsessive-compulsive disorder (OCD). About 20-25% of children and up to 53 percent of adults with ADHD may have anxiety or depression. People with anxiety disorders often worry excessively about many things and may feel edgy, stressed out, tired and tense and have trouble getting restful sleep.

5. Mood Disorders

Approximately 38 percent of adults with ADHD have a coexisting mood disorder. Extreme changes in mood characterize mood disorders. Children with mood disorders may seem to be in a bad mood often. They may cry frequently or become irritable with others for no apparent reason.

Some children with ADHD will go on to develop mania. Up to 20 percent of people with ADHD may show bipolar disorder symptoms, a severe condition involving periods of mania, abnormally elevated mood and energy, followed by episodes of clinical depression.

The bipolar child may alternate between feelings of importance with periods of depression or irritability. If left untreated, bipolar disorder can damage relationships and lead to job loss, school problems, and even suicide.

6. Autism Spectrum Disorder (ASD)

Autism spectrum disorder is a condition related to brain development that impacts how a person perceives and socializes with others. It's estimated that two-thirds of individuals with ADHD also show features of ASD. Studies show that between 30 and 50% of individuals with ASD also show symptoms of ADHD.

7. Tic Disorder or Tourette Syndrome

Tics disorder involves sudden, rapid, recurrent, involuntary movements, or vocalizations. Tourette Syndrome is a much rarer but more severe tic disorder. Tourette syndrome is a neurological condition that causes various nervous tics and repetitive mannerisms.

Some people with tic disorder or Tourette syndrome may often make noises, clear their throats frequently, snort, sniff, or bark out words, and make repetitive movements such as flinching or blinking. Sometimes, these tics can be made worse by ADHD medication.

Not many children have Tourette syndrome, but many people with Tourette syndrome also have ADHD. Less than 10 percent of those with ADHD have tics or Tourette Syndrome, but 60 to 80 percent of those with Tourette Syndrome have ADHD.

8. Substance Use disorders

Research suggests that youth with ADHD are at increased risk for very early cigarette use, followed by alcohol and then drug abuse. Cigarette smoking is more common in adolescents with ADHD. Youth with ADHD are twice as likely to become addicted to nicotine as individuals without ADHD. Adults with ADHD have higher rates of smoking and more difficulty in quitting.

9. PANDAS or Pediatric Autoimmune Neuropsychiatric Disorder Associated with Streptococcal Infection

PANDAS is an autoimmune condition triggered by strep throat infections, which disrupt a child's normal neurologic activity. Symptoms usually appear abruptly overnight.

With PANDAS, the immune system produces antibodies, intended to fight an infection, but instead, it mistakenly attacks healthy tissue in the child's brain, resulting in inflammation of the brain.

Children with PANDAS frequently get misdiagnosed with attention deficit hyperactivity disorder (ADHD), autism, bipolar disorder, or OCD that is unrelated to any infection.

10. Celiac Disease

One Italian study reported *significant improvement in ADHD symptoms in ADHD kids with Celiac disease on a gluten-free diet for 6 months*. The researchers tested 67 people with ADHD for celiac disease. Study participants ranged in age from 7 to 42. A total of 15 percent tested positive for celiac disease. That's far higher than the incidence of celiac in the general population, which is about 1 percent.

Another study investigated the incidence of ADHD symptoms in people with newly diagnosed celiac disease. It looked at 132 participants, ranging from toddlers to adults. The study showed that a gluten-free diet improved ADHD symptoms substantially in about six months after starting the diet.

As a registered dietitian and holistic health coach, I focus on helping parents identify the different triggers of ADHD symptoms in their children. *Most children with ADHD have multiple triggers and causes, including genetics, environmental toxins, food intolerances, and nutrient deficiencies*.

While medication and behavior modification certainly help with "symptom control," *diet and lifestyle modification can bring about long term symptoms relief* because it gets to the root causes of the symptoms.

From that perspective, I've found that *dietary strategies to be the cornerstone of a successful natural ADHD treatment program*.

After all, *which child does not deserve proper nutrition?*

Why is My ADHD Child Always Hungry?

Parents often ask "Why is my child always hungry?"

Or some kind of variations like, *"he's always asking for snack right after dinner*? Or *"waking up in the middle of the night binging on junk food,"* Or *"I find candy wrappers in her bedroom"*.

People often wonder if ADHD affects appetite.

The answer is "yes" and "no".

Yes because the *dopamine reward center of the brain is messed up in ADHD*. This reward center also regulates appetite and hunger. So, naturally, it is affecting appetite.

No because *ADHD is not the only reason why your child's appetite is whacked*.

The answer is really simple.

In adults, we call it "cravings". In kids, we call it "hungry" because that's what your child always say, "mom, I'm hungry".

We know when you have cravings, your body is telling you something is missing, usually some kind of nutrients, but we always ended up eat junk food with empty calories, then we end up binging because our body did not get what it needs.

The way to look at this is really simple.

When we're hungry, our body needs energy.

When we're thirsty, our body needs hydration.

When we have cravings, our body needs vitamins and minerals.

Just that simple.

So when your child say, "mom, I'm hungry". They are hungry for nutrients - things like vitamins, minerals and antioxidants.
They're not starving for energy, so giving them more goldfish crackers or granola bar will not help.

Some of you may even notice that your child craves salt as well. That's definitely a sign of mineral deficiency.

In fact, nutrient deficiencies are very common in children with ADHD. This's been proven by scientists over and over again.

The most common nutrient deficiencies in children with ADHD are magnesium, zinc, iron, vitamin D, vitamin Bs and omega-3 fatty acids.

There are **2 *main underlying causes for nutrient deficiencies in children with ADHD*** making them always hungry and always asking for or sneaking food.

1. Poor Food Choices.

This comes no surprise because everyday I see parents trying their best to give their children what they think is the best. But what I see is they're feeding them what food manufacturers think is best for their families.

Every kid that I see, their snacks include a repertoire of processed crackers, cookies, chips, puffs, cakes, candies, chocolates, fruit snacks, sugar-loaded yogurt. Breakfast are always sugary cereals, poptarts, granola, bagels, pancakes, waffles, etc. Lunch and dinner are usually chicken nuggets, hot dog, pizza, etc.

Where are the real foods? What vitamins and minerals do you get from these food?

These are so-called "kid food" or "kid-friendly food".

Why do kids have to have their own food like dog food and cat food?

Shouldn't kids be eating the same *human food* as their parents?

I know parents are trying their best to feed their families.

But these food are cheap, convenient, "fun", "kid-friendly" and "healthy" according to the TV commercials.

Do you really know what's in these food? How much does these food affect your child's ADHD symptoms?

Not only do these processed food provided no nutritional values, but they are also loaded with processed sugar and high fructose corn syrup, which the ADHD brain has difficulty processing. When the ADHD brain is fed a carb-loaded diet and cannot use their sugar for energy, it sends distress signals to the body that it's starving.

2. Poor Digestion

This is a little more complicated concept. ***Most people assume everything that we eat are 100% broken down into the basic units*** of amino acids, glucose, fatty acids, vitamins and minerals.

But the digestion process is quite complicated and for many people, especially kids with ADHD, this process is not efficient.

When food you eat are not properly broken down, our body cannot pull the nutrients from the food.

When food are not being digested properly, it can actually hurt the intestine and create tiny little holes, where undigested food can end up in our blood stream and trigger allergic reaction and inflammation.

For some kids, the allergic reaction and inflammation caused by poorly digested food one of the many causes behind their lack of focus (brain fog in adult term), hyperactivity (restlessness) and mood swings.

Poorly digested food also changes the intestinal environment causing gut bacteria imbalance.

Poor digestion can also be caused by nutrient deficiency. ***Your body needs a lot of different nutrients to make stomach acid, and digestive enzyme to break down food.***

Keep reading. Step 2 of the *Eat to Focus Program*, we'll address this issue.

The Scary Truth About Untreated ADHD

ADHD is among the most debilitating disorders to live with when left untreated. It is more than just a neuro-developmental disorder. It's a huge public health concern because untreated ADHD can adversely affect every aspect of one's life and longevity. ADHD can reduce life expectancy by as much as 13 years, but its risk is reversible.

The negative consequences of untreated ADHD go beyond the inability to focus and forgetting and losing things, as some of the consequences can change the course of someone's life.

Because of the inherent lack of self-regulation and impulsiveness, it frequently results in poor judgment, poor self-care, and high-risk behaviors. A person with ADHD is more likely to say or do things without thinking them over, resulting in both emotional and physical harm toward one's self and others.

Children with ADHD can have a hard time paying attention in class and may not learn everything they're taught. They may fall behind in learning or get poor grades.

A study showed that up to 58% of children with untreated ADHD failed a grade in school. In another study, 46% of children with ADHD had been suspended from school. And as many as 30% of adolescents with untreated ADHD fail to complete high school, compared with 10% of those without ADHD.

People with untreated ADHD are more likely to engage in substance abuse and cigarette smoking. It is also more common for children with ADHD to start abusing alcohol during their teenage years.

In a study of 538 adolescents, substance use was reported in 63% of the 165 girls and 56% of the 79 boys with ADHD symptoms. In another study involving 946 adolescents aged 15 years in New Zealand, alcohol-related problems were reported in 23% and illicit drug use in 21% of the 82 subjects who had been diagnosed with severe attention-deficit behaviors at age eight years.

Another study looked at 334 college students (mean age of 21 years). The incidence of tobacco and marijuana use was significantly higher in the 76 students (23%) who reported a history of ADHD than in students without a history of ADHD.

In regards to health, 38% of young adults with untreated ADHD have unplanned pregnancies or have caused an unplanned pregnancy, compared with 4% of those without ADHD. And seventeen percent of young adults with ADHD have contracted a sexually transmitted disease, as opposed to 4% of those without.

The epidemic of traffic fatalities has also been linked to untreated ADHD. Driving is the most dangerous activity that teenagers do, and car accidents are the leading cause of death among young adults in North America.

The research found that drivers with ADHD had a 36 percent higher risk of crashing than peers without ADHD. With driving performance seriously impacted by inattention, and impulsiveness, young drivers with untreated ADHD have two to four times as many motor vehicle crashes as their peers without ADHD.

ADHD also interferes with personal relationships, negatively affect family cohesiveness, reduce the chances of personal success and satisfaction, and put healthy marriages at risk. Those with untreated ADHD are twice as likely to divorce as their treated or typical peers.

Children with untreated ADHD may have trouble making or keeping friends as they may not know how to share toys, take turns, or play with others nicely. These can result in social isolation, low self-esteem, and depression.

Despite all these, ADHD is one of the most treatable mental health disorders. With proper diagnosis and proven treatments, people with ADHD may live a normal functional life.

When you correct the underlying causes of the ADHD symptoms appropriately, the body begins to heal, and your child begins to learn new skills to achieve their personal goals, improve relationships, meet deadlines, avoid accidents on the road, and regain confidence and happiness in life.

CONVENTIONAL ADHD TREATMENT APPROACH

Conventional medicine looks at ADHD as a biochemical disorder caused by dysfunctions in the brain, specifically a deficiency in certain neurotransmitters.

A medical doctor will probably tell you that the ADHD brain is deficient in two neurotransmitters - dopamine and norepinephrine, which are chemical signals that the brain uses to communicate between brain cells.

The conventional treatment protocol consists of behavior-modification programs and pharmacotherapy with stimulant drugs. These stimulants work by increasing both dopamine and norepinephrine.

This process is the basis or rationale for using stimulant medications that supposedly changes (or hijacks) the brain (control center) chemistry to force the reduction of ADHD symptoms.

Both dopamine and norepinephrine are involved in many essential body functions, such as sleep, moods, hunger, etc.

Dopamine is associated with mood, risk-taking, impulsivity, and reward. Norepinephrine is believed to moderate attention, arousal, and mood.

That's why there are horrible side effects, such as personality change and mood swings with ADHD medications.

If you're lucky, your doctor will prescribe behavioral modification along with ADHD stimulant meds. Unfortunately, most patients only get the medication part.

While these treatment approaches often improve symptoms, complete resolution of symptoms is rare, and cure is infrequent.

How do ADHD Medications Work?

Currently, the first line of treatment for ADHD is medication. As soon as a child is diagnosed with ADHD, the pediatrician starts medication right away.

There is also evidence that shows these medications may cause stunt growth. And up to 30% of patients do not respond to stimulants.

I'm not against medication. I genuinely believe there are kids with ADHD out there who NEED the medicine to calm down enough to learn life skills to manage their ADHD symptoms and correct their brain biochemistry. Then, they can slowly wean from the medication.

Most ADHD medications are stimulants that increase the level of the neurotransmitters, dopamine, and norepinephrine by inhibiting their clearance. Both dopamine and norepinephrine are essential to brain chemical signals for proper brain function.

There are mainly two types of ADHD medications: stimulants and non-stimulants.

Stimulants are the most commonly prescribed medications to treat ADHD in children. They've been used to treat ADHD since the 1960s and are some of the most researched of all drugs used with kids and adults. Studies show they work well in about 70 to 80 percent of patients.

For many children with ADHD, stimulant medications increase concentration and focus while also reducing hyperactive and impulsive behaviors.

ADHD stimulant medications work by *increasing the amounts of dopamine and norepinephrine*, which are both neurotransmitters or brain chemicals for signaling. These medications target the brain's reward system that involves the brain chemical, dopamine, which plays a crucial role in motivation, pleasure, attention, and movement.

Stimulants increase dopamine levels in the brain by slowing the "recycling" process. There is concern that when brain chemicals in the brain are artificially boosted, it may cause a depletion in the rest of the body, resulting in potential neurotoxicity of amphetamine.

Some of these medications start working within 30 minutes of taking. Others take up to 60 to 90 minutes before they kick in.

Stimulant ADHD medications include amphetamine (Adzenys XR ODT, Evekeo), amphetamine/dextroamphetamine (Adderall and Adderall XR), dextroamphetamine (Dexedrine, ProCentra, Zenzedi), dexmethylphenidate (Focalin and Focalin XR), lisdexamfetamine (Vyvanse), and methylphenidate (Concerta, Daytrana, Metadate CD, and Metadate ER, Methylin and Methylin ER, Ritalin, Ritalin SR, Ritalin LA, Quillivant XR).

When stimulants don't work, or patients are experiencing unpleasant side effects, non-stimulant medications are used.

Non-stimulant ADHD medications include a few antidepressants and blood pressure medications, which help to improve concentration and help with impulse control.

Non-stimulant ADHD medications include amitriptyline (Elavil), desipramine (Norpramin, Pertofrane), imipramine (Tofranil), nortriptyline (Aventyl, Pamelor), or other tricyclic antidepressants, bupropion (Wellbutrin), escitalopram (Lexapro), sertraline (Zoloft), and venlafaxine (Effexor).

Is ADHD Medication Safe?

Parents worry about caffeine stunt growth, and I've never in my 18 years professional career see a child with stunt growth because of caffeine.

But I can look at the growth chart of any children with ADHD and can tell you exactly when the child started ADHD medications.

Caffeine is being used as a lung surfactant in brand new premature babies in the neonatal intensive care unit (NICU) every day. It's a common practice in all NICUs everywhere. So giving children caffeine is not a new or unusual practice.

So why can't we try some caffeine or other natural stimulant first before ADHD medications?

If there's no other option, and ADHD medications are the only choice. That's a different story.

ADHD medications can reduce the symptoms of hyperactivity, inattentiveness, and impulsivity in children and adults with ADHD. However, these medications come with horrible side effects and dangerous outcomes that you might want to think twice.

That's why ADHD medications should be only for children with severe cases of ADHD that are interfering with social life and school work.

As much as 70% of patients on ADHD medication report side effects, such as loss of appetite, weight loss, stunt growth, headaches, stomach ache, sleep disorder, mood swings, irritability, and facial tics zombie-like state, and personality change.

I have many parents complain to me that the ADHD medications turn their children into a "zombie" or "not being themselves." Some of my kid patients would tell me that "I don't like my personality when I'm on the medicine."

Long term use of such medications may increase the body's tolerance and dependence on these drugs, which may lead to a higher risk of drug addiction in adulthood.

Strattera may cause suicidal thoughts and actions in some children and teenagers, especially if your child has bipolar disorder or depression in addition to ADHD.

This is a tough choice. Do I want a hyper child? Or do I want a suicidal child?

Or a dead child?

In March of 2006, an FDA panel reported that 11 sudden cardiac deaths in children taking Ritalin and Concerta between 1992 and 2005. Both medications contain the stimulant methylphenidate. They also reported 13 sudden cardiac deaths among children taking the amphetamine-containing stimulants Adderall and Dexedrine.

Hmmm...

Take your time to rule out other possibilities, weigh your options, and get your child's input in the decision-making process.

Trust your instincts and do what feels right to you and your child. Don't let anyone — be it your physician or the principal at your child's school — pressure your child into medication if you're not comfortable.

Remember: medication isn't the only treatment option.

Starting ADHD medications should always be personalized and closely monitored by a trained psychiatrist (not a psychologist or your pediatrician).

I am a trained and experienced specialist in pediatric nutrition, and I worked with many highly qualified and experienced pediatric subspecialty doctors. Therefore, I know the value of the care that a specialist provider versus a general practitioner provides.

FUNCTIONAL ADHD TREATMENT APPROACH

Conventional ADHD treatment usually consists of behavioral accommodations and medication, with stimulant medication most commonly being prescribed.

Current ADHD medications target only a few biochemical pathways to manipulate neurotransmitters to suppress behaviors. However, it does not completely remove the root cause of the problem, whatever it is. That is the reason why many children with ADHD do not respond well to the medications.

A simple analogy to illustrate the idea of medication for ADHD is stepping on a piece of broken glass. You can take loads of pain killer to numb the pain on your foot, but as long as the piece of broken glass remains in your foot, the pain remains.

Same as in the case of ADHD, you can try all kinds of ADHD medication to mask the symptoms. But if the root cause remains, and so will the symptoms.

Unfortunately, the root cause of ADHD is not as clear-cut or obvious as the piece of broken glass. Some detective work is required in most cases, along with some experimentation.

ADHD medications don't cure ADHD. They are only for symptoms relief. ADHD medications are "boo-boo bandaid" for the problem without treating the underlying causes.

I see children with ADHD frequently, mostly for just two reasons why these patients are referred to me. These children are either failure to thrive due to the anorexic side effects of ADHD medications or those newly diagnosed with ADHD, and parents want to try the "natural way" or "the diet" first.

More parents are aware and concerned about the side effects and long-term use of conventional ADHD medications and are increasingly interested in alternative treatment options.

Complementary and alternative ADHD treatments offer families many options, including dietary modifications, nutritional supplementation, herbal medicine, and homeopathy that do not have the same side effects as convention ADHD medications.

Alternative ADHD treatment can also be an excellent complementary treatment to conventional ADHD treatment to maximize treatment outcome or as an alternative treatment option for milder cases.

In some cases, it may help to reduce the amount of medication needed and, thus, reduction in side effects.

The functional approach focuses on identifying the underlying root causes and imbalances to develop an individualized treatment plan specific for the patient. This approach results in significantly better patient health outcomes and satisfaction.

ADHD is a diagnosis based only on reported and observed symptoms and behaviors. And the conventional treatment is based on symptoms. All kids and adults with the same symptoms or ADHD get the same medication.

Current conventional medicine ignores that many underlying causes cause ADHD behaviors and that each individual is different.

Even though ADHD is defined by the narrow set of signs and symptoms, there could be multiple underlying causes.

This simple fact explains why a treatment that works for your friend's child does not work for your child.

Most children have multiple causes, which explains why you may find one treatment that works well but does not have complete symptoms resolution because there may be another cause or causes that still need to be corrected.

While medication and behavior modification certainly help with "symptom control," diet and lifestyle modification can bring about long-term symptom resolution because it gets to the root cause of the symptoms.

After all, which child does not benefit from proper nutrition?

Other less talk about symptoms of ADHD include diarrhea, constipation, skin rash, eczema, asthma, food allergies, etc. are clues to what's going on in your child's brain and body. These symptoms are clues to your ADHD detective work.

6 Possible Root Causes of ADHD No One Talks About

The diagnosis of ADHD is based on the presence of ADHD symptoms, specifically lack of focus, hyperactivity, impulsivity and poor memory, etc. that are impacting school and social life.

However, when it comes to treating ADHD, conventional treatment continues to focus on these symptoms.

But did you know *there are many causes of ADHD*?

Everyone who has ADHD has the *same ADHD symptoms*, but each person's *underlying causes are different*. That's why there's no one diet or supplement or anything that works for everyone with ADHD.

It's the same reason why ten patients with breast cancer who receive the same treatment will have ten different treatment results.

Another way to look at it is by comparing it to headaches. Everyone who has a headache is called "a headache sufferer."

But each person has a headache for a different reason. It could be signs of *dehydration, hunger, brain tumor, concussion, sinus allergy, and even a brain aneurysm*.

Would you be okay if your doctor gives you a pain killer for your headache if the cause of your headache was a brain tumor or brain aneurysm?

However, the causes of ADHD in children are not black and white, as there may be multiple causes.

I have many parents who told me how they restrict sugar and red dye because they cause their kids to become "hyper."

So does merely eating sugary food cause ADHD?

Possibly.

However, the causes of ADHD is a lot more complicated than just eating too much sugar. It's a lot more than that, but this could be one reason.

There is no genetic testing or blood test or brain scan to confirm the diagnosis of ADHD.

The diagnosis is all based on behaviors observed by parents, teachers, and care providers. And it's all subjective, based on individual opinions.

The best way to get a proper diagnosis and proper treatment plan is a thorough evaluation by a developmental pediatrician and/or a pediatric psychiatrist.

I know adults who are diagnosed with ADHD and started on ADHD meds. But when asked further, this individual sleeps only 4 hours a night and deals with a lot of life stressors.

Is ADHD the right diagnosis? Would you take ADHD medications for your lack of sleep? Or is behavior counseling more appropriate to help cope with stressors, which would solve insomnia, which will lead to better sleep quality?

Let's look at some causes of ADHD that can be corrected by changing what you eat.

- ADHD Brain
- ADHD Gut
- Hidden Food Allergies
- Poor Nutrition
- Genetic Defects
- Environmental Toxins

1. ANATOMY OF THE ADHD BRAIN

I remember going to a parent orientation at my daughter's school at the start of the school year. And one of the topics discussed was the expectations of a 7th grader.

Basically, it's the school way to tell us, parents, to chill and don't expect too much from our 7th graders, because their "prefrontal cortex" is still developing.

The way I look at *ADHD is that attention and memory are like other developmental skills, such as crawling,* walking, talking, etc.

Every child masters each skill at their own pace, and we have a set range of time when these skills are learned.

If you look at ADHD the same way you look at when your child ate his/her first food, spoke his/her first word, took the first steps, etc., you'll better understand some of the symptoms of ADHD.

We'll talk about the 4 Surprising Facts about the ADHD brain and how it differs from the neurotypical brain.

1. The ADHD Brain is Smaller

A study published in The Lancet Psychiatry looked at the brain scans of over 3,000 people between the ages of 4 and 63, both with and without ADHD.

The study concluded that those with ADHD had smaller brain volumes compared to people without ADHD. Interestingly, the differences are more prominent in children with ADHD and not as much in ADHD adult brains, which means individuals with ADHD likely catches up with brain growth as they get older.

That's good news.

Children with ADHD typically have smaller prefrontal lobe (10% smaller), which is the brain region responsible for reasoning, planning, solving problems, controlling attention, impulsivity, executive function (ability to plan and organize), focus and complete task.

When the prefrontal cortex isn't functioning correctly, you'll see more fidgeting and acting on impulses.

2. The ADHD Brain is Behind or Delayed

Another imaging study done by researchers at the National Institutes of Health's (NIH) National Institute of Mental Health (NIMH) showed that the ***brain of children with ADHD is three years behind in maturity and with typical development as children without ADHD***.

This means the ADHD brain's development is behind the actual age. So a ten-year-old child with ADHD might be functioning at the level of a seven-year-old, which is why he or she has the attention span and impulsivity of a seven-year-old.

The delay in ADHD was most prominent in regions at the front of the brain's outer mantle (cortex), which is essential for controlling thinking, attention, and planning.

Some babies start walking at seven months, some walk after 13 months. Some speak early, and some need more help with speaking.

My daughter had a speech delay as a toddler. She did not utter her first word until 18 months of age. And her first word was "apple," which was at the time her favorite food. She needed speech therapy for the first few years of her life.

The ***good news is that the ADHD brain is not small forever***. It eventually catches up with peers. That's one reason why ADHD symptoms tend to decrease or disappear in adolescence or adulthood.

3. The ADHD Brain is Low on Brain Chemicals.

The *ADHD brain also has a lower level of dopamine*, a neurotransmitter (or brain chemical) associated with reward, desire, and motivation. A deficiency in dopamine is linked to a lack of motivation and poor motor control.

There are two possible causes of a deficiency in dopamine:
1. The body is not able to make enough due to nutrient deficiency and defective pathways
2. Defects in receptors genes and transporter proteins of neurotransmitters

Receptors are the final destinations, where the dopamine attaches to in the brain. If there is a problem getting these neurotransmitters to their destination, the brain cannot function correctly and results in ADHD symptoms.

4. The ADHD Brain Does not Like Sugar

Parents ask me all the time, "Why does my child crave sugar all the time?"

While it may not seem obvious that problems with attention, hyperactivity, and impulsivity could be related to food cravings, but there is a connection between the ADHD brain and sugar cravings.

Glucose powers all cells in the body. Glucose increases cortical activation in reward-control areas. However, the ADHD brain cannot process glucose very efficiently compared to non-ADHD brains.

That means less energy is available for the attention center in the prefrontal cortex, which we already know is smaller and behind in kids with ADHD.

The ADHD brain uses 8% less glucose than the non-ADHD brain. When the brain does not get enough glucose, it sends out distress signals to the body to demand more glucose, and that's how cravings for sugar or sweets start.

Many people indulge in sugar-rich food, such as candies, cookies, soda, fruit juices, and other highly processed "junk foods" because these food can be quickly converted to glucose for the brain to use.

Research shows that low levels of dopamine in ADHD are related to cravings for sugar and other highly processed carbohydrates.

Sugar and other high carb foods boost dopamine levels in the brain, leading kids and adults with ADHD to crave them more often when dopamine levels are low.

Since kids with ADHD have chronically low levels of dopamine, they are more likely than neurotypical kids to crave and eat sugary or carbohydrate-heavy foods.

High fructose corn syrup is the most potent stimulus for dopamine release because of the fructose molecules. The more table sugar or sucrose you eat, the more dopamine you release.

Over time, this leads to a reduction in dopamine receptors and dopamine receptor-mediated signaling.

Regular sugar consumption may lead to a "sugar addiction" that involves behaviors similar to those seen with classical drug addiction.

The dopamine response from regular sugar consumption is entirely different than the dopamine response when we eat a piece of yummy steak.

While the yummy steak also release dopamine, but it's mostly due to the novelty of the food, and the release of dopamine decreases with subsequent exposure to the food.

You know how you eat the same food three days in a row?

However, when kids with ADHD eat sugar daily, the dopamine response to sugar slowly decreases, and you need more and more sugar to get the same "sugar high."

In response, sugar cravings continue to increase due to their addictive effects. However, over time, the frontal lobe becomes less sensitive to natural rewards, resulting in the development of behaviors such as overeating seen in kids and adults with ADHD.

It is no wonder that those with ADHD struggle with eating disorders. Each time they self-medicate with sugary food, their brain enjoys a surge of dopamine and energy burst that improves attention and short-lived calmness.

As a result, most kids with ADHD gravitate toward a diet consists of mainly highly processed food, which also causes unstable blood sugar fluctuations that produce some of the crazy behaviors seen in kids with ADHD, such as anger outburst, aggression, emotional mood swings or meltdowns.

You know, "Hangry"?

The feeling you have when you are HUNGRY and ANGRY at the same time?

Yes…your child is HANGRY!

I know you just feed your child.

The problem is the food.

Highly processed snacks, such as crackers, chips, cookies, granola bars, fruit snacks, etc. all these causes blood sugar fluctuations or roller coasters.

When you eat carbs or sugar, your body reacts with producing insulin, which ushers the sugar into cells for use as energy.

However, when you eat carbs or sugar in large quantities, your body overreacts with making too much insulin, forcing the sugar into cells too fast. This results in a sudden drop in blood sugar, which many people are familiar with as the "sugar crash."

This "sugar crash" is responsible for many mood swings and temper tantrums.

The other issue with this scenario is that the insulin remains high until your next carb-loaded meal/snack, which keeps the insulin high all day. When insulin level is up, it blocks the body from using fat as energy.

The body is supposed to use stored fat and protein between meals for energy. It's the exact reason why we don't starve to death overnight when we're sleeping for long hours and not being fed for 8 hours. Now your blood sugar level tanks and you can't use fat for energy. You're stuck with no energy source.

That's when your child throws a raging tantrum demanding more goldfish crackers or tear the house down.

If your child does not process sugar well for energy, then a sugar- and carbohydrate-rich diet consist of mostly processed carbs can do more harm than good as we've just discussed.

Knowing that the ADHD brain is behind and does not play well with sugar, the best ADHD diet should focus on brain-building nutrients and avoiding sugar, especially fructose.

The ADHD brain defects account for only a small percentage of ADHD cases. Therefore, we need to consider other possible factors that might cause or predispose individuals to develop ADHD.

And that's the ADHD Brain …it's smaller and on average three years behind a neurotypical brain, and it's also low on brain chemical, called dopamine.

2. ANATOMY OF THE ADHD GUT

Does your ADHD child suffer from *stomach pain, bedwetting, fecal incontinence, diarrhea, loose stool, or constipation*?

Does your ADHD child also have *food allergies or intolerance, asthma, ear infections, and unexplained skin rash*?

Or does your child crave milk, cheese, sugar, bread, noodles, pasta, crackers, or any carbs?

Chances are all these symptoms are related and can all be traced back to the gut imbalance.

Even though conventional ADHD treatment often focus on treating what's happening in the brain, but most of the explosive and aggressive behaviors in ADHD kids seem to stem from the gut.

When the gut balance is disrupted and out-of-balance, mental and physical health issues, such as anxiety, depression and even cancer can happen.

In recent years, scientists have discovered the connection between gut bacteria and many psychiatric and neurodevelopmental disorders, such as autism spectrum disorders, ADHD, depression, anorexia nervosa, and Rett syndrome.

They found that brain chemical imbalances, often seen in people with ADHD, may have started in the gut, causing more aggressive and explosive symptoms.

Scientists learned that the gut is talking constantly with the big brain (aka central nervous system that includes the brain and spinal cord). They talk to each other continuously through the hormonal, immune, and nervous systems.

The gut bacteria do not live for free in our intestines. They do pay rent by *making precursors (ingredients) that the big brain can use to produce brain chemicals,* such as dopamine, noradrenaline, and serotonin, that help to calm the ADHD brain.

Based on what scientists know so far about the *gut-brain connection, they concluded that our gut is possibly the second brain.*

Digestive *symptoms were found to be related to behavioral problems, including social withdrawal, irritability, and repetitive behaviors.*

Autism spectrum disorder (ASD) and ADHD are both early-onset neurodevelopmental disorders. They are both umbrella terms that cover a wide range of abnormal behaviors and developmental disorders.

ADHD is characterized by inattentive, hyperactive, and impulsive behavior whereas the key symptoms of ASD include social deficits, communication deficits, and stereotypical behaviors.

Children with ADHD and ASD also share similar behavioral symptoms such as anger outbursts, impulsivity, aggressiveness, agitation, and emotional meltdowns. Indeed, research shows that ASD and ADHD frequently exist together.

Studies have shown that *children with autism and ADHD experience more stomach and digestive issues such as constipation, diarrhea, and sensitivity to foods* six to eight times more often than children who are developing typically.

Did you know 75% of the body's immunity is in the gut? It is host to over 1,000 different species of bacteria, known as the 'gut microbiome. Every individual has his or her own microbiome make-up, like fingerprints.

These bacteria help digest and absorb nutrients and move food through your intestine. They also keep your intestine lining secure and intact to keep foreign intruders out of your system.

The interaction between the gut and the brain can be illustrated with the vascular system of a tree.

The roots in the ground draw up vital nutrients and water from the soil and communicate with other plants. Those nutrients are then brought up to the tree's body, fortifying and building the trunk and giving the tree what it needs to sprout new leaves, which then gather lights, another energy source.

In the same way, nutrients from the food we eat are absorbed through our intestines (tree roots). We rely on those nutrients to fuel our brains.

While our brains take up only 2% of our total body weight but it uses 20% of energy we take in. Therefore, nutrients play a huge role in how our brain functions on a daily basis.

The gut is lined with 100 million nerve cells and makes up part of the enteric nervous system or ENS. When your baby is growing in the womb, the ENS and CNS grow from the same tissue and remain connected via the vagus nerve. The two systems mirror each other and produce the same brain chemicals, such as dopamine, serotonin, and acetylcholine, etc.

The nerve cells in the gut work in very similar mechanism as the brain. The gut is made up of the same neurons as the CNS, and a network of bacteria that form the microbiome, which is a unique as our fingerprint.

If you feed your gut with junk food, you're also fueling your brain with junk fuel.

Frequent Antibiotics & Acid Suppressant Use

Candida or yeast overgrowth and bacterial overgrowth may be the causes of the digestive issues your kids with ADHD are dealing with.

Don't believe it? Keep reading…

76% of new cases of bacterial infection are in children who had recently been prescribed antibiotics. Frequent use of antibiotics for treating ear infection in children *not only kills the bacteria that cause the infection, but it also kills the good bacteria living in the gut*.

So don't demand antibiotics if your doctor says your child doesn't need them. Nearly 50% of antibiotics are inappropriately prescribed.

20% had taken stomach acid-reducing drugs (Aciphex, Dexilant, Nexium, Prevacid, Prilosec, and Protonix), which is linked to increased risks for *C. diff* infection.

Studies also suggest the majority of people who take the popular class of stomach acid-reducing drugs known as proton pump inhibitors (PPIs) don't need them.

These two classes of drugs could potentially cause yeast and bacterial overgrowth, which can result in hyperactivity, anger, irritability, hyper-excitability, mood, memory, poor attention, sleep problem, and inappropriate behaviors.

Candida Yeast Overgrowth

Does your child have frequent ear infections needing antibiotics? Does your child also crave sugar?

Candida is a fungus, a form of yeast that lives in your mouth and intestines in small groups. Surprisingly, with all the bad reputation, candida, fungus, or yeast do have a few benefits.

It helps with digestion and absorption of nutrients. It also makes some essential vitamins and nutrients for the human host, while the human host provides them with a lovely warm home in the intestines.

But when the good bacteria are wiped out by antibiotics or not fed well with a high fiber diet, or there's too much sugar to feed the yeast, the gut's delicate ecosystem is damaged. Then, yeast and other harmful organisms take over.

Candida is an opportunistic fungus, which means it thrives or multiplies freely when the opportunity opens up, such as a high sugar diet. These little guys become trouble when there are too many of them.

Candida produces toxins that can leak from the gut into the brain and block the prefrontal cortex, which we now know is smaller in the ADHD brain. This results in hyperactivity, anger, irritability, moodiness, poor memory, poor attention, sleep problem, and inappropriate behaviors.

A high-sugar, low-fiber diet can trigger yeast or candida overgrowth, impaired immunity, use of drugs like antibiotics, birth control pills, estrogen, and steroids, and psychological stress.

Children are particularly vulnerable to these kinds of insult because of their immature immune system.

Telltale signs of candida overgrowth are addictive behaviors towards sweets and sugar. Like the saying, "I'll *kill for a cookie*," and calms down completely after eating sugar.

Bacterial Overgrowth

Does your child also have persistent diarrhea that does not go away? Has your child been on antibiotics and/or stomach acid suppressants?

Your child's aggressive behaviors may also be the result of a clostridium difficile infection.

A new study shows the potentially deadly diarrhea bug *Clostridium difficile*, or *C. diff*, is spreading among children in the community.

The waste product of c. diff is 3-(3-hydroxyphenyl)-3-hydroxypropionic acid or HPHPA for short. HPHPA *blocks the conversion of dopamine to norepinephrine in the brain.* This result in too much dopamine in the brain, which can cause extreme aggressive behaviors, anxiety, rage, and agitation.

When the body cannot convert dopamine to norepinephrine and epinephrine, other brain chemicals are affected. This imbalance may cause permanent damage to the brain, adrenal glands, and sympathetic nervous system.

If your child's aggressive behaviors become worse when starting ADHD medications that boost dopamine, they may most likely have a c. diff infection.

The gut needs a combination of both good and bad bacteria to do all its job correctly. When the intestinal gut balance is disrupted and out-of-balance, mental and physical health issues, such as anxiety, depression, and even cancer, can happen.

And that's the ADHD gut …it's imbalanced because of yeast overgrowth and possibly bacterial infection as well.

3. HIDDEN FOOD ALLERGIES IN ADHD

If your child has eczema, asthma, and frequent ear infection, there's a very likely chance that your child's ADHD symptoms may be related to food sensitivities.

Children with ADHD are more likely to have allergy (immune-mediated) disorders like food allergy, asthma, and atopic dermatitis (eczema).

What comes to your mind when you hear the words "food allergies"?

The picture is the scene of Will Smith in "Hitch" after he ate an appetizer with shrimp, which he's severely allergic to. His whole face and ears literally swell up.

That's the kind of allergic reaction people often think of. People often associate food allergies with only physical manifestation. However, many food allergies and intolerances manifest itself in more subtle behavioral ways.

Can you think of an incident when your child suddenly acts unlike himself or herself after eating certain foods?

Like he or she started acting silly after eating certain foods? Or he or she throws a raging tantrum for crackers, and after having the crackers, he or she would calm down?

I hear stories like these all the time.

One time, after I picked up my daughter from school, and she started talking non-stop, which is not her usual self. Later I found out she had pepperoni at the after school program. We don't usually eat pepperoni in our house.

Children with ADHD often have hidden food allergy or intolerance. I use the word "hidden" because these allergies or intolerances are difficult to identify.

People are often completely unaware that they have a food sensitivity. A negative blood or skin test for food allergies does not mean that a child is not sensitive to certain foods.

Most of the time we don't even know they exist because when we think of food allergy, we are thinking of the very obvious ones, like someone who is an allergy to seafood, and ate something with shrimp, and within minutes reacted with full-body hives, facial swelling, itching mouth, and throat, etc.

However, these are not what we see in most children with ADHD. Their reactions are a lot more subtle and slow. The food reactions we often suspect in children with ADHD or autism are food intolerances.

Food intolerance and food allergy share many similar signs and symptoms, such as diarrhea, vomiting, runny nose, nasal congestions, hives, rash, etc. However, they are very different physiologically.

Before we go further, I would like to clarify the difference between a true food allergy and food intolerance because many people are confused between the two.

Food Allergy vs. Food Intolerance

We often refer to any food reaction as a food allergy. However, most of these reactions are food intolerances instead of allergies.

True food allergy triggers an immediate immune response, usually involving the immunoglobulin E (IgE). IgE-mediated response activates a cascade of systemic reactions, involving multiple organ systems. That is why this is the more severe form of food intolerance and will show up on the blood allergy test.

Fatal peanut allergy falls into this category. Even a tiny amount of the offending food can cause an immediate, severe reaction or anaphylactic shock, a life-threatening allergic reaction.

Anaphylaxis is characterized by systemic responses, such as difficulty breathing due to swelling of the airway, hives, and itching, flushed or pale skin, weak and rapid pulse, dangerously low blood pressure, nausea/vomiting, or diarrhea, dizziness or fainting.

An anaphylactic event requires emergent medical treatment, and delay of treatment may result in death. People with severe food allergies are usually prescribed and "epi" epinephrine pen that they carry around in case they eat or come in contact with their allergen by accident.

With a true allergy, the offending food needs to be avoided altogether, especially in young children.

Food allergies are common in the first years of life. With every repeated exposure to the offending food, the immune system becomes better in attacking that allergen, which means the response will become more and more intense each time the body is exposed to the allergen.

Most children usually outgrow their allergies by 4 or 5 years of age. However, repeat exposure may prevent or delay the time to outgrow the allergy.

On the other hand, food intolerance usually does not involve the immune system, and reaction also comes on a lot slower – usually couple hours after eating the food, and even up to 48 hours – and more subtle presentation. The individual usually can tolerate a small amount of the offending foods without much adverse effect.

Symptoms of food intolerance are generally less dangerous, less obvious, and appear very subtly and slowly. That's why that trouble food is seldom identified.

Some common signs and symptoms include nausea, vomiting, abdominal cramps, constipation, diarrhea, asthma, eczema (atopic dermatitis), etc.

True story here…it took me years to finally figure out I have a gluten intolerance. I'll tell you my gluten story another time. For now, I would like to focus on your child.

Food intolerances may also result in symptoms frequently seen in ADHD and autism, such as "brain fog," absentmindedness, anxiety, agitation, fatigue, etc.

Causes of Food Intolerance

There are many causes of food intolerance or food allergy. There may be a lack of enzymes to thoroughly and efficiently digest a food. Or it may be a leaky gut, which allows partially digested food into the bloodstream aggravating immune responses.

Lactose intolerance is a perfect example.

People frequently thought they are "allergy to milk." Let me clarify it here...

If you are "allergy to milk," you CANNOT have any milk product at all – milk, cheese, yogurt, and anything made with or contains dairy ingredients.

If you are "lactose intolerant," on the other hand, you can tolerate a small amount of milk with your morning cereal or coffee, enjoy some yogurt, cheese, or ice cream without a problem. But you definitely cannot drink a lot of milk by itself. If you have 10/10 stomach cramps or have to "sprint" to the bathroom after drinking milk, you have "lactose intolerance." Those are not allergic reactions.

In lactose intolerance, the body does not produce enough lactase (an enzyme that breaks down lactose into glucose and galactose). Lactose or milk sugar causes osmotic diarrhea.

Delayed food intolerance can also trigger ADHD symptoms through a systemic inflammatory process.

Poor Digestion and Food Reactions

Your child may be eating the food without *getting the nutrients because the food he or she eats is not adequately broken down*, digested, and absorbed.

Food eaten needs to be digested correctly to be absorbed and used by the body. *Undigested food rots and ferments in the intestine causing gas and bloating and, of course, upsetting the gut bacteria balance.*

And *a small piece of partially digested food may enter the bloodstream and trigger an allergic reaction and systemic inflammation*.

Your body only knows amino acids, fatty acids, glucose, vitamins, minerals, electrolytes, and other natural biochemical compounds. It does not recognize pieces of organic chicken or grass-fed beef.

Food needs to be adequately broken down and digested not to trigger an allergic reaction.

Your child may also be *sensitive to food additives*, such as preservatives, food coloring, monosodium glutamate, sodium benzoate, etc., which is the basis of the Feingold diet, introduced by Dr. Benjamin Feingold in 1975 to treat children with ADHD.

Autoimmune conditions, such as type 1 diabetes and Celiac disease, may trigger adverse reactions to foods. We'll talk about Celiac disease later as there's a strong relationship between Celiac disease and ADHD.

Cow's Milk and Gluten Intolerances in Children with ADHD

When a child cannot eat and absorb nutrients properly, he or she cannot grow, learn, explore, or develop properly.

Every child benefits from proper nutrition, but when children with special needs are given additional nutrition support, the changes in their behavior, mood, learning, sleeping, and development are amazing.

The most common food sensitivity in kids with ADHD and autism are *sensitivities to casein and gluten*.

Casein is a protein found in milk and milk products such as cheese, butter, yogurt. Gluten is a protein found in wheat, barley, and rye.

People on the autism spectrum and have ADHD may not be able to properly digest casein and gluten due to a lack of enzymes.

In normal healthy digestion, casein is broken down into casomorphin and gluten into gliadorphin. These peptides are then further broken down into individual amino acids, which then enters the bloodstream.

When these proteins are not properly digested, the casomorphin and the gliadorphin can leak into the bloodstream before being further broken down. Once these proteins enter the bloodstream, they can get through the blood-brain barrier to the brain.

Both of these proteins act like opioids, such as heroin and cocaine, and bind to the same opioid receptors in the brain.

And this peptide morphine affects your child's behavior, just like cocaine and heroin.

Yes, your child is drugged on food.

In susceptible children, ***these undigested proteins cause fatigue, aggression, irritability, moodiness, anxiety, depression, and brain fog.***

Besides, the undesired mental effects, these proteins also trigger silent allergic reactions, such as ***allergic shiners (dark circles under eye), colic, runny nose, ear infections, eczema, belly pain, bad breath, and insomnia***, etc.

Eliminating these offending protein from the diet is the only solution or treatment option.

A child with high levels of casomorphin may have intense cravings for milk products (ice cream, yogurt) and may even become irritable when he or she doesn't eat these types of foods.

If your child shows addictive behaviors around dairy and wheat products, such as milk or cheese and bread, pasta, noodle, crackers, there's a great chance your child with ADHD or autism may not be breaking down milk and gluten protein properly.

Parents often describe their children as very irritable and cranking when not having these items, and then calm down into a sweet angel after eating them.

There is a simple urine test that can measure levels of both casomorphin and gliadorphin. The test determines sensitivities even when a patient has no IgE or IgG allergic reactions to these foods.

This is one of the reasons why ADHD medication or supplements or a clean diet, or a vegan diet does not work for every child because the issue is not in the brain. And also one of the reasons why other ADHD treatment does not work. It's because the cause is in the digestion.

So now we know your child most likely has a food intolerance and not a food allergy. This explains why the food allergy test almost always comes back clean.

The allergy tests that your pediatrician use – Radio-AllergoSorbent Testing (RAST) and skin prick test – only identify allergic reactions caused by the immunoglobulin E (IgE). Remember, the reactions we see in food intolerance do not involve the immune system. Thus, RAST and skin prick will pick up nothing.

The oral challenge is the gold standard of food allergy testing. In this case, you remove gluten and casein from your diet for at least two weeks or until you see symptoms improve, then reintroduce one food back at a time. If symptoms worsen with reintroduction, you know your child is intolerant to that food.

The best we have is observation and keeping a detailed food and behavior log. Sometimes you may be able to pinpoint a few foods that your child reacts to.

Inside *Eat to Focus*, you'll learn how to eliminate these foods from your child's diet to calm him or her down.

Some parents would swear that their child will act up after every time their child eats or drinks anything with red coloring.

You've probably noticed when your child's eczema worsens with eating dairy products. Or your child starts acting silly and unable to focus after eating a lot of wheat products or processed food.

Many studies are showing the association between Celiac disease and ADHD. In one study, researchers tested 67 people with ADHD for celiac disease. Study participants ranged in age from 7 to 42. A total of 15% tested positive for celiac disease, which is far higher than the incidence of celiac in the general population, which is about 1%.

A gluten-free diet significantly improved ADHD symptoms in patients with celiac disease in this study. For people with gluten sensitivity, studies show that gluten may play a role in ADHD symptoms. However, it's less clear.

And that's the common hidden food allergies in ADHD…gluten and casein sensitivity, and *it's mostly due to poor digestion and poorly digested food.*

4. MALNUTRITION IS COMMON IN KIDS WITH ADHD

When we think of malnutrition, we often think of pictures showing starving kids in Africa. Or your parents used to tell you, "eat all your food, kids are starving in another country."

Even though malnutrition is still a significant public health issue in many developing countries, *overweight and obesity are becoming serious threats to children in the United States*.

Overweight and obesity are forms of malnutrition. Malnutrition (both under- and over-nutrition) during childhood may affect the health and performance of children when they become adults.

Malnutrition is associated with poorer IQ levels, cognitive function, school achievement, and more behavioral problems *such as attention deficits, and emotional instability.*

Children in the US have better access to food, but that does not mean they have better nutrition or better health. According to the Center for Disease Control (CDC), between 2015-2016, *nearly 1 in 5 school-age children and young people (6 to 19 years old) in the United States have obesity*.

Children in the US eat too many empty calories from processed foods that are lacking in essential nutrients, causing excessive weight gain and nutrient deficiencies.

There are decades of research to support the *strong relationship between ADHD and obesity*. Remember, in the Anatomy of the ADHD Brain, we talked about *how low dopamine levels and effects of sugar can cause sugar addiction and overeating in people with ADHD?*

A *person with ADHD is four times more likely to become obese* than someone who does not have ADHD.

There are hundreds and even thousands of biochemical reaction pathways in the body that are going on constantly to sustain the function of the body. *Every single one of these pathways and reactions requires at least one mineral and vitamin that acts as a catalyst to turn on that pathway.*

When there is a mineral or vitamin deficiency, some biochemical reactions are being affected, resulting in the body not functioning correctly, and you have "dis-ease."

When we look at our anemic food supplies – *genetically modified organisms or GMO products* that are not suitable for human consumption, *manufactured food* that's been stripped off of essential nutrients, over-farming causes *mineral depletion in the soil* from which our fruits and vegetables come from, you see how your body can become deficient in nutrients over time.

And do you see why getting proper nutrition is difficult?

We, human beings, can only thrive on simple, pure food and a clean environment.

Unfortunately, all these are affecting our children. Children with ADHD are found to be deficit in magnesium, zinc, iron, omega-3 fatty acids, vitamin Bs, vitamin D, and many others.

Eating a healthy diet alone is not enough to correct nutrient deficiencies. In step 2 of the *Eat to Focus Program*, we also look at a few ADHD supplements to start to correct the most common nutrient deficiencies in kids with ADHD.

Premature Babies and ADHD

Babies who are born too soon or weigh too little at birth are about three times more likely to develop ADHD than full-term, healthy-weight infants.

When babies are born premature, they did not have the opportunity to fully develop and build up their store of nutrients before coming to this world. Therefore, many of them are born, not only malnourished, compared to their term peer, but they're also fighting to get whatever nutrition they can to catch-up growing.

We keep premature babies on high calories, high fat, high protein, high calcium, and high phosphorus diet to help them keep up with their growing needs to give them another chance outside mom's comfortable womb.

Even with this knowledge of what they need, their nutrition still often come short because their tender premature body is not ready for an outside source of nutrition.

Necrotizing enterocolitis (NEC) is common in premature babies. The only way to minimize NEC is with exclusive breastmilk, but breastmilk is also too low in calorie, protein, and minerals for premature babies.

To give them the right amount of nutrients to meet their needs requires a large volume of breastmilk that's often too much for their body to handle. We fortify breastmilk to maximize nutrient intake.

Another challenge of premature infants is that many develop oral aversion from many orally intrusive procedures or lack of opportunity to learn to eat by mouth. With oral aversion, feeding becomes difficult and limited.

Many premature babies continue to suffer many disabilities and delays despite all the medical and nutrition interventions early in life.

Essential Fatty Acid Deficiency in ADHD

Multiple studies have shown that children with ADHD have very low blood levels of omega-3 fatty acids, *an average of 38% lower than children without ADHD*. Children with *low dietary omega-3 intake are 31% more likely to be diagnosed with ADHD*.

Lower levels of omega-3 fatty acids are also associated with autism, ADHD, dyslexia, apraxia, depression, and anxiety. Low DHA (docosahexaenoic acid) levels are associated with more defiant and hostility, mood swings, and learning difficulty.

Omega-3 fatty acids make up about 8-10 percent of brain tissues. It is the major component of myelin sheaths on nerve cells. Myelin is the fatty coating on nerve cells.

The *myelin sheaths insulate nerve cells (imagine electrical wiring) to ensure the smooth, uninterrupted transmission of impulses, preventing misfiring of nerve impulses*.

When your child is little, he or she is making many of these myelin sheaths in the brain. That's why the brain doubles in weight by the age of two years old.

This is also the reason why babies and young child needs to be on a high-fat diet.

A low-fat diet is harmful to children. *Low essential fatty acids level causes the outer covering myelin layer to degenerate*, resulting in brain cells making fewer brain chemicals, which controls mood and behaviors.

Omega-3 fatty acids also protect the brain by controlling the low-grade inflammation or oxidative stress.

The low essential fatty acid level also causes the cellular receptors for dopamine to form incorrectly, resulting in lower dopamine levels and more symptoms of ADHD. This is one of the causes of low dopamine levels we discussed previous chapter.

Our ancestors ate a diet of 2:1 ratio of omega-6 to omega-3 thousands of years ago. Today's a typical Western diet is 20:1, which *is excessive in omega-6 and deficit in omega-3 fatty acids*.

This comes to no surprise as the standard Western diet consisted of mostly mass-produced animal protein, vegetable oil, and trans fats in many processed foods.

We eat way too much omega-6 fatty acids in the form of processed foods. To correct this, you need to *reduce dietary omega-6 intake while increasing your dietary omega-3 intake to achieve the optimal 4:1 ratio*.

The good news is you can cheat a little here. Researches and studies have shown that *omega-3 fatty acids supplementation can improve ADHD symptoms*, such as hyperactivity, inattentiveness, aggression, anxiety, impulsiveness, and learning difficulties.

The omega-3 fatty acid is one of the nutrients most studied in children with ADHD. And therefore, omega-3 fatty acid or fish oil supplements is always the first supplements I start most patients on. Almost every single patient responded well to fish oil.

There are two kinds of essential fatty acids: omega-3 and omega-6. Most modern diets have plenty of omega-6, but omega-3 is relatively scarce.

The three main omega-3 PUFAs are eicosapentaenoic acid (EPA), docosahexaenoic acid (DHA), and alpha-linolenic acid (ALA). EPA and DHA are mainly found in marine oils (fish, krill, seal, whale). ALA is in some vegetable oils, such as flaxseed oil.

Micronutrient Deficiencies in ADHD

Does your child seem hungry all the time, crave sweets, and salty foods? Does your child also have issues with anxiety and moodiness?

Micronutrient deficiency may be the cause.

Micronutrients are nutrients that the body needs only in tiny amounts. However, they all play essential functions in the body. These include all vitamins, minerals, and antioxidants.

Micronutrients are used as cofactors in enzymatic reactions and play a significant role in metabolism, neurotransmission, cognitive function, immune function, and detoxification.

Minerals and vitamins are essential for many body functions, such as cell metabolism, making brain chemicals, growth, and development. Our bodies cannot make their own minerals and vitamins, so they must come from food or supplementation.

Because of *modern agricultural practices* such as over-farming, fertilizers, and soil erosion, our soil is tragically depleted in minerals and vitamins. Besides, when *food is processed*, it is further stripped off of essential micronutrients. Plus, the *stress we encounter in our daily lives* increases the metabolism of many vital vitamins and minerals as well.

You can't get a brain cell to fire appropriately when there are not enough minerals in the body, just like you cannot conduct electricity through distilled water.

Your body is indeed a machine because it runs on electricity. That's why having enough electrolytes and minerals is so important.

The three most common mineral deficiencies in kids with ADHD are *magnesium, zinc, and iron*. The four most common vitamin deficiencies in kids with ADHD are *vitamin B6, vitamin B12, folate, and vitamin D*.

Magnesium Deficiency in ADHD

Many studies show that magnesium deficiency is common in children with ADHD. One study showed up to 72% of children with ADHD have a magnesium deficiency. There was a significant correlation between hair magnesium, total IQ, and hyperactivity.

Another study even showed 95% of children with ADHD with magnesium deficiency.

Magnesium is one of the most abundant minerals in the body and is involved in over 300 metabolic reactions, including cellular energy generation, nucleic acid production (DNA, RNA), and protein synthesis.

Magnesium deficiency is associated with impulsiveness and hyperactivity, sensitivity to loud noises, insomnia, depression, anxiety, irritability, restlessness, panic attacks, fatigue, both salt and carbohydrate craving, and carbohydrate intolerance.

Remember, we talked about the ADHD brain does not do well with carbs earlier?

Over the last century, magnesium content has been progressively declining in our food supply, thanks to all the highly processed foods that floods our supermarkets, modern fertilizers, and over-farming.

A diet high in genetically modified grains and legumes, refined sugars, soft drinks, and caffeine all deplete magnesium. It is estimated that about 50% of Americans of all ages do not eat enough magnesium from their diet.

People used to consume an average of 450-500mg of magnesium a day from whole real food alone, today we only average 175-225mg a day, if any.

Testing for magnesium is complicated and unreliable as 90% of the body's magnesium is stored in the bones and the rest in soft tissues. Less than 1% of total magnesium is in blood serum, and these levels are kept under tight control by the kidneys.

That's magnesium…

Zinc Deficiency in ADHD

Zinc deficiency is also common in ADHD. In a recent case-control study, *70% of children with ADHD between the ages of 6 and 16 were zinc deficient.* Those with lower hair zinc levels had the worst hyperactivity, inattention, oppositional, and impulsivity scores.

In another study of 118 children with ADHD, those with the lowest blood levels of zinc had the most severe conduct problems, anxiety, and hyperactivity as rated by their parents.

Multiple studies have confirmed that zinc levels are lower in children with ADHD, but the extent of zinc deficiency is inversely correlated with symptom severity in those with ADHD. Researchers have also linked zinc deficiencies with several other neuropsychiatric disorders, including ADHD.

It is difficult to assess the zinc level in the body, as most blood tests are inaccurate. However, if your child has frequent or chronic diarrhea, he or she is losing zinc from diarrhea.

Zinc is an essential trace mineral needed in the *central nervous system and makes vital brain chemicals*, such as dopamine, norepinephrine, serotonin, and GABA.

Zinc is required to synthesize dopamine, norepinephrine, and serotonin and enhance GABA, one of our primary inhibitory/relaxation brain chemicals. It is also an essential factor in the metabolism prostaglandins, and for maintaining brain structure and function.

Many lifestyle factors can deplete zinc, causing a deficiency or imbalance as well.

Zinc deficiency is more common in children who eat a minimal diet of processed food. A diet depleted of zinc-rich food, such as red meat, seafood, and chicken, may result in low zinc and high copper imbalance.

ADHD symptoms sometimes worsen with puberty due to the higher metabolic demand for growth during puberty. And this can deplete zinc and cause copper excess.

Also, *an increased stress hormone, such as cortisol, can block zinc activities.* The demanding practice and game schedule of a competitive athlete can also deplete zinc stores. This is more so if the athlete is a vegan as well.

Environmental toxins, such as Bisphenol A (BPA) and phthalates found in everyday plastic products, bind and deplete zinc levels in the body as well.

Symptoms of Zinc Deficiency in ADHD

1. Picky eating habits with a strong sense of taste and smell perception may be signs of zinc deficiency. Low zinc level block sensation of taste and smells and make meat tastes repulsive. Parents would usually notice things like, "Junior can tell when we buy a different brand of chicken nuggets," or "We can't hide anything in Junior's food because he always can taste it the difference" or "Junior always complain the food tastes or smells funny."
2. Allergies are commonly a result of too much copper as a result of zinc deficiency, which weakens the immune system.
3. The digestive problem, especially diarrhea, which is a common symptom of zinc deficiency.
4. Sleep disorder may be a result of zinc deficiency as well since zinc is needed to make melatonin.

Zinc deficiency may result in poor or loss of appetite, diarrhea, impaired immune function, poor or retardation of growth, delayed sexual maturation, eye or skin lesions, delayed wound healing, taste abnormalities, and mental lethargy.

These signs and symptoms of zinc deficiency are not very specific and may be associated with other health conditions. Therefore, it is essential to seek medical advice if your child shows any of the above signs and symptoms.

Low zinc levels can interfere with the effectiveness of ADHD medication. Studies show that kids on both Ritalin and zinc supplements showed better ADHD symptoms control with lower Ritalin doses.

How Does Zinc Help ADHD?

In a 2004 study, children aged 6 to 14 were randomized to take 150mg zinc sulfate or a placebo daily for 12 weeks. Those who take the actual zinc supplement had significantly reduced symptoms of hyperactivity, impulsivity, and impaired socialization.

Another similar study in 2009, when over 200 children were randomized to 15 mg of elemental zinc a day or placebo for ten weeks, those taking zinc supplements saw significant improvement in attention, hyperactivity, oppositional behavior, and conduct disorder compared to the placebo group.

In a more recent study, *children treated with a daily dose of 40mg of elemental zinc as zinc sulfate for 12 weeks showed significant improvement in scores on hyperactivity, impulsiveness, and impaired socialization scales* than the children given a placebo.

Iron Deficiency in ADHD

Iron deficiency is common in kids with ADHD. Many researches show that both low serum iron and low ferritin (storage iron) were associated with ADHD symptoms, such as more hyperactive, inattentive, and impulsive. Serum iron is the iron swimming in the bloodstream, and ferritin is iron stored in cells.

Studies showed almost *92% of kids with ADHD have a low ferritin level.* Kids with iron deficiency are 67% more likely to have ADHD. The lower the levels are, the more severe the ADHD symptoms and cognitive impairment. *Children with an iron deficiency do poorly in math and language skills.*

Low iron level is also associated with sleep disorder, depression, low IQ, autism spectrum disorder, anxiety, bipolar disorder, delayed development, and mental retardation, which are all common in kids with ADHD.

Iron is needed in making dopamine and melatonin. Kids with low ferritin also seem to need a higher dose of ADHD medication to calm down.

Restless leg syndrome is also common in kids with ADHD. Children with low ferritin levels are also more like to suffer from restless leg syndrome (RLS), which is a condition that causes an uncontrollable urge to move your legs. It usually happens in the evening or nighttime while sitting or lying down.

Well, it seems like most kids with ADHD have the urge to move.

Iron deficiency can also be the result of eating too many dairy products. We all know dairy products are rich in calcium. When you overeat dairy products, there's also a lot of calcium in your diet. Calcium and iron are absorbed the same way by the body. When there's too much calcium in your diet, the calcium is being absorbed instead of the iron, and that causes iron deficiency.

Don't start the iron supplement just yet. Iron is one of those supplements that you don't want to mess with because too much iron can be dangerous.

I always check iron levels before starting patients on iron supplements. And the choices of supplements also is based on the results of the iron profile.

Iron supplements can help improve ADHD symptoms, such as impulsivity control, hyperactivity, and aggression, but it may also help make ADHD medication more effective. So less medication is needed and fewer side effects.

Having adequate iron also prevent lead poisoning, which is a possible cause of ADHD symptoms.

Vitamin B6 Deficiency in ADHD

Vitamin B6 (pyridoxine) is an essential vitamin necessary for more than 60 biological processes in a healthy human body. It holds many big jobs that affect your mood, appetite, sleep, and thinking. You need it to fight off infections, turn food into energy, and help your blood carry oxygen to all corners of your body. While it's rare to run low of it, you can't afford to do so.

The body converts vitamin B6 from the food we eat into pyroxidal-5-phosphate (PLP), an enzyme that is used to release energy from carbohydrates and break down proteins. PLP is also used in the production of essential brain chemicals.

How does Vitamin B6 Help with ADHD?

The body needs vitamin B6 to make the brain chemicals affected in children with ADHD, including serotonin, dopamine, and norepinephrine. PLP is necessary for the conversion of DOPA into dopamine (the missing brain chemical in ADHD) and conversion of glutamate (the exciting brain chemical) to GABA (the calming brain chemical).

The level of vitamin B6 available determines how much of the brain chemicals are made. Even a mild vitamin B6 deficiency can result in substantially low production and less GABA and serotonin being made. As a result, sleep and behavior are being affected.

Besides its involvement in brain chemical productions, *vitamin B6 also has a direct effect on immune function and plays a role in brain glucose regulation*.

Pyridoxal-5'-phosphate is also associated with inflammation, and levels of pyridoxal-5'-phosphate are down-regulated as a function of more severe inflammation, potentially as a consequence of pyridoxal-5'-phosphate's role in the metabolism of tryptophan. This role is particularly crucial as *inflammatory processes may contribute to dementia and cognitive decline*.

Symptoms of Vitamin B6 Deficiency

Children with ADHD and autism have lower conversion rates to PLP, the active form of vitamin B6. Therefore, supplementing with PLP is more appropriate and readily available for use by the body.

Inside the body, the naturally occurring glycosylated forms of vitamin B6 in fruits and vegetables must be converted by the liver to the active form the body needs. *People with impaired liver function, celiac disease, older adults, and children with autism and ADHD have decreased ability in converting vitamin B6 into its active forms.* Therefore, supplementing vitamin B6 in its active form, is more appropriate and readily available for use by the body.

Vitamin B6 deficiency can cause irritability, impaired alertness, depression, cognitive decline, dementia, autonomic dysfunction, convulsions, seborrheic dermatitis, peripheral neuropathy with numbness and tingling in hands and feet, brain fog.

WHAT STUDIES AND EVIDENCES SAY?

In one study, 40 children with clinical symptoms of ADHD were followed for up to 8 weeks during a trial of magnesium-vitamin B6 (Mg-vitamin B6) regimen.

Children from the ADHD group showed significantly lower magnesium levels than children in the control group (n = 36). In almost all cases of children with ADHD, being on the Mg-B6 regimen for at least two months significantly reduced clinical symptoms of hyperactivity and aggressiveness and improvement attention in school.

Besides, the Mg-B6 regimen also significantly increased magnesium values in the group of children with ADHD. Unfortunately, when the Mg-B6 treatment was stopped, ADHD symptoms reappeared just a few weeks, along with a decrease in magnesium values.

Vitamin B12 Deficiency in ADHD

Vitamin B12 deficiency is common in children with autism spectrum disorder (ASD) and attention deficit hyperactivity disorder (ADHD).

A study published in 2019 looked at the serum level of vitamin B12, folate, and homocysteine in 118 children (48 children diagnosed with ADHD, 35 children diagnosed with autism spectrum disorder (ASD), and 35 healthy controls).

The study found that children with ASD had the lowest levels of vitamin B12, and also the highest levels of homocysteine, followed by children with ADHD. Healthy children in the control group have the highest level of vitamin B12 and the lowest homocysteine level.

Vitamin B12 and folate play essential roles in the development, differentiation, and functioning of the central nervous system. They are involved in the methionine-homocysteine pathway, responsible for the methyl groups required for DNA and protein synthesis.

Low vitamin B12 levels may increase the level of homocysteine, which is known to be a powerful excitotoxin. Its by-products may cause nerve damage and disrupt the production of brain chemicals, which are essential for the structural integrity of the brain.

Symptoms of Vitamin B12 Deficiency

Vitamin B12 deficiency is usually the result of poor intestinal absorption due to intestinal surgeries or intestinal disorders, or inadequate dietary intake, such as a vegetarian or vegan diet, which restricts animal products.

Vegans who do not eat any animal products, including eggs and dairy, are more likely to develop vitamin B12 deficiency because of their restrictive diet. Ovo-lacto-vegetarians usually consume enough B12 through eggs and dairy products.

Vegans obtain vitamin B12 from dietary supplements and fortified foods, such as fortified breakfast cereals, fortified soy products, fortified energy bars, and Brewer's yeast.

Occasionally, certain medications may increase its metabolism in the body.

Deficiencies in vitamin B12 and folate levels cause changes in the homocysteine level, which might be related to depression, mood disorders, psychotic disorders, and obsessive-compulsive disorder.

Recently, some studies have reported deficiencies in vitamin B12 and folate (vitamin B9) in patients diagnosed with ASD and ADHD and the beneficial effects of those vitamins for some of the associated ASD and ADHD symptoms.

Vitamin B12 deficiency affect the nerves (numbness, tingling, tremors, balance problems) and the mind (depression, brain fog, memory loss, mood swings, and, in rare cases, dementia, hallucinations, and psychosis).

Taking folic acid (folate) or eating a lot of folate-containing foods without adding B-12 can actually mask the symptoms of a developing B-12 deficiency.

Take folate will keep your blood count normal even if your vitamin B12 is falling, and the folate will not protect your brain and nervous system. Your symptoms of numbness, tingling, balance problems, and emotional issues will continue unchecked.

How Does Vitamin B12 Help ADHD?

All of the B vitamins work together synergistically to support critical functions in the brain. All of the B-complex vitamins are co-factors to each other – that is, they help each other to be absorbed and utilized properly by the body.

In studies, B-complex vitamins have been shown to reduce hyperactivity symptoms and increase serotonin in children with ADHD, resulting in calmer, happier children. And children taking methylcobalamin showed increased executive function.

Preliminary studies suggest that vitamin and micronutrient supplements may reduce emotional liability, aggression, and oppositional behaviors in children with ADHD and ASD. Studies also support the use of vitamin B12 supplements for improving symptoms of depression in people deficient in this vitamin.

Vitamin B12 supplementation may also help improve sleeping likely because methylcobalamin enhances the body's supply of melatonin.

Vitamin D Deficiency in ADHD

Several studies have found a link between vitamin D deficiency and neurodevelopmental disorders, such as ADHD. Vitamin D plays a vital role in healthy brain development and function.

In a case-control study in Qatar, 1,331 children diagnosed with ADHD (ages 5–18) were matched with children without ADHD. There was a statistically lower level of 25-OH vitamin D in the ADHD group compared with healthy controls. 19.1% of children with ADHD *vs.* 12.7% of healthy controls had 25-OH vitamin D levels of less than ten ng/mL, indicating severe deficiency.

In a cross-sectional study, a group in Turkey measured 25-OH vitamin D in children (ages nine ± 2.2 years old) diagnosed with ADHD ($n = 60$) and compared these to a healthy control group. The ADHD group had statistically lower levels of 25-OH vitamin D.

Another recent study found that vitamin D deficiency was seen more in children with ADHD than in the control group. In children with ADHD, the average vitamin D level was 16.6 ng/ml; in contrast, in children without ADHD, it was at 23.5 ng/ml.

What is Normal Vitamin D Level?

According to a committee of the Institute of Medicine, someone with a serum 25(OH)D concentrations <30 nmol/L (<12 ng/mL) are at risk of vitamin D deficiency. And you are potentially at risk for *inadequacy* at levels between 30–50 nmol/L (12–20 ng/mL). A level ≥50 nmol/L (≥20 ng/mL) is considered sufficient. Serum concentrations >125 nmol/L (>50 ng/mL) are associated with potentially adverse effects.

25-hydroxyvitamin D (25-OH) is considered the best measure of vitamin D status. It reflects both vitamin D made in the skin and vitamin D eaten from food and supplements.

Serum 1,25-dihydroxy vitamin D, the active form of vitamin D, is not a reliable measure of vitamin D because it has a short half-life. And it may remain normal even in deficiency.

Symptoms of Low Vitamin D Deficiency?

In children, vitamin D deficiency causes rickets, a disease characterized by bone tissue failure to mineralize, resulting in soft bones and skeletal deformities properly.

Rickets was first described in the mid-17th century by British researchers. In the late 19th and early 20th centuries, German physicians noted that eating 1–3 teaspoons of cod liver oil daily could reverse rickets.

Certain medical conditions, such as kidney disease, liver disease, intestinal malabsorption, can result in vitamin D deficiencies. So are people with darker skin pigmentation, limited sun exposure, and taking anti-epileptic drugs.

Vitamin D deficiency is also common in someone following diets that exclude animal protein products, such as vegans.

The symptoms of vitamin D deficiency are often very subtle. And many people don't even realize they are deficient in vitamin D. Some of the symptoms of vitamin D deficiency may include:
- Fatigue or tiredness
- Bone and muscle pain
- Low mood and energy
- Anxiety
- Irritability
- Weight gain
- Hair loss

Low vitamin D levels in children have also been associated with allergies, asthma, and eczema. In adults, it can lead to osteoporosis or osteopenia (soft bones).

How Does Vitamin D Help with ADHD?

Vitamin D is a steroid that has been shown in both animal and human studies to be essential for healthy brain development.

Vitamin D receptors and the enzyme responsible for creating the active form of vitamin D, are everywhere in the central nervous system (spine and brain).

They are found in the brain cells of brain regions that have been associated with defects resulting in ADHD.

There is also evidence that shows vitamin D deficiency during development can affect the dopamine system, which is the defective brain area in the ADHD brain.

In animal models, vitamin D has been shown to be associated with the production of tyrosine hydroxylase, the rate-limiting enzyme for dopamine synthesis.

4 Benefits of Vitamin D for the ADHD Brain:

- Increases dopamine and norepinephrine levels, which reduces the negative symptoms of ADHD
- Increases production of acetylcholine, which helps you to maintain focus, concentration, and memory
- Encourages the growth of nerve cells for memory storage and executive function
- Increases the release of serotonin, which helps with depression and seasonal anxiety disorder

5. GENETIC DEFECTS

Does your ADHD child's mood and behavior worsen after taking a regular multivitamin or even eating fortified cereals?

A genetic defect may be the cause.

A study of 40 kids with ADHD found that the ADHD group had significantly more MTHFR gene mutation than the control group.

The MTHFR gene is needed to make the enzyme that turns folic acid or folate into its bioavailable form, methylfolate, which then converts amino acids for a variety of the body's functions, including the production of serotonin and dopamine.

Folic acid supplementation may be harmful to a child with ADHD if the child has this specific genetic mutation. Folic acid is a synthetic product and does not occur naturally in nature. Folic acid is NOT the same as folate, which is vitamin B9.

The body normally converts folic acid and folate into methyltetrahydrofolate (MTHF), the bioactive form of the B vitamin that your body needs for a variety of normal functions.

However, this process is frequently defective in kids with ADHD.

Folic acid is the synthetic version often found in supplements and processed foods. The body can only utilize folic acid after it is converted to methyfolate. Therefore, folic acid does not help with ADHD.

MTHFR (methylenetetrahydrofolate reductase) is the name of both a gene and an enzyme in the human body that tells the body how to make the enzyme that turns folic acid or folate into its bioavailable form, methylfolate.

The methylfolate then converts amino acids for a variety of the body's functions, including the production of serotonin and dopamine. This reaction is needed for the converting the amino acid homocysteine into methionine (another amino acid).

The body uses methionine to make proteins and other essential compounds, such as chemical messengers (serotonin, norepinephrine, epinephrine, dopamine, and melatonin). These brain chemicals have potent effects on mood, energy, sleep, digestion, muscle and nerve function, memory, and cognition.

MTHFR gene defects have been associated with several health issues, including mood disorders like depression, anxiety and schizophrenia, and neurobehavioral disorders like ADD/ADHD and autism.

If the MTHFR gene is mutated, it cannot make the enzyme correctly, which disrupts serotonin and dopamine production, critical players in ADHD, autism, and mood disorders.

Activated folate, a.k.a. methyltetrahydrofolate (MTHF) is an important part of something called the methylation cycle. This metabolic cycle is involved in neurotransmitter production, detoxification processes, and the regulation of inflammation.

MTHFR also helps in the process of detoxification in the body. When it's not working properly, heavy metal and minerals can reach dangerous levels or become imbalance, which can cause hyperactivity, mood disorders, and so much more.

Symptoms of MTHFR Gene Mutation

If not treated, MTHFR mutations can cause folic acid to buildup in the blood and causes mood and behavioral disorders worse.

The buildup of folic acid may be the reason why some kids with ADHD have sensitivities or rare reactions to medications, and even supplements. It also explains why mood and behavior can *worsen when your child takes a regular multivitamin or even eats fortified cereals*.

Symptoms of MTHFR mutation vary among individuals and depending on the type of mutation. Some people may have no symptoms at all. Others may have more severe complications like increased risk for heart disease, sluggish detox, miscarriages, and more.

People usually do not know that they have an *MTHFR* mutation unless they experience severe symptoms or undergo genetic testing.

Children with MTHFR gene mutations may be at increased risk for ADHD, learning disabilities, autism, or autoimmune disorders. However, just because one inherits the mutation does not necessarily mean they will have all the problems.

Having one or two *MTHFR* mutations can slightly increase the levels of homocysteine present in the blood. Homocysteine is an amino acid that the body produces by breaking down dietary proteins. High levels of homocysteine can damage blood vessels and lead to blood clots. People who have high homocysteine levels tend to have low levels of vitamin B12.

Symptoms of homocysteinemia due to *MTHFR* mutations include:

- abnormal blood clotting
- developmental delays
- seizures
- microcephaly (small brain)
- poor coordination
- numbness or tingling in the hands and feet

6. ENVIRONMENTAL TOXINS EXPOSURE AND ADHD

Environmental toxins are everywhere. We live in a giant pool of pollution every day. Children with autism and ADHD or other developmental disorders seem to be more susceptible to environmental toxins.

The first thing we wake up in the morning, we brush our teeth. There is hexavalent chromium (aka chromium-6, does the name Erin Brockovich ring a bell?) in water, then the fluoride and sodium lauryl sulfate and artificial sugar in toothpaste.

Then, your first cup of joe made with the same chromium-6 water, artificial sugar (of course, it's the healthier choices for sweetening, and non-dairy creamer (check the ingredient list on the label – can't find much familiar English words).

It's time to go. You step out of your door and take a deep breath of fresh air. Sorry, it's not fresh air, but exhaust-filled air from the rush-hour traffic. Don't worry. There are even more chemicals waiting for you in your office – flame retardant on almost everything, formaldehyde, toluene, xylene, styrene, benzene (just to name a few) in carpets.

Lunch is a meal of processed food filled with meat from corn-fed cattle, treated with antibiotics and growth hormones. The greens from your supposedly healthy toss salad are genetically modified to deter disease and infection and also loaded with pesticides fresh from the soil.

Well, I guess I should stop before I get myself too depressed to eat for the rest of my life. My point here is toxins are everywhere, and we cannot avoid all of them altogether. You'll have to move to Mars to avoid all these.

Each one of us is made differently. Some of us have an excellent immune and detoxification system to get rid of these toxins efficiently from the body. Others have a so-so system to do the trick.

There's been an increase in the incidence of ADHD, autism and other developmental disorders over last 20 years, which somehow coincide with the astronomical expansion of the processed food industry, the increasing use of food additives, growth hormones and antibiotics in lives stocks, and other chemical used in industries in the name of boosting food production.

Although evidence shows that ADHD runs in the family, families share the same environment and food supply. These include prenatal substance exposures, heavy metal and chemical exposures, nutritional factors, and lifestyle/psychosocial factors.

How much of it is genetics, and how much is environmental?

Heavy metals, such as lead and mercury, are on top of the list of environmental toxins. These have been proven to affect brain growth and development in children.

Manmade food additives and preservatives interfere with the body's hormonal system, causes systemic inflammation and changes brain chemistry and brain functions.

Most people's idea of environmental toxins, they're thinking about the air and water we breathe, but it's everything that we interact with every day - air, water, food, medicine, furniture, receipts, people, etc.

1. Lead

Lead is one of the most studied environmental toxins in relation to mental disorders, such as conduct disorders, the intelligent quotient (I.Q.), and ADHD.

We now know a great deal about how lead affects the brain, including disruption of signaling in the prefrontal cortex and striatum.

Lead's effects on children's I.Q., ADHD, and conduct problems, as well as physical health, have been of concern for decades.

Many studies using different methods between 2005 and 2015 had confirmed that the blood lead level was associated with ADHD even at concentrations in the 0.5 to 3.0 µg/dL range, after control for other factors.

The mean lead level in these studies was well below the *Centers for Disease Control and Prevention* recommended safe level of 10 µg/dL.

Therefore, a "safe" level of lead for children should be "undetectable" on the current testing equipment. Any detectable level should be monitor and further investigated.

Lead is found in paint in building built before 1978, lead pipes in old buildings, antique furniture, and paint in toys imported from other countries, which does not have the same regulations as the United States.

Most children in the U.S. (about 70%) are exposed to lead through lead paint in older houses, schools, and other buildings built before 1978, from surrounding soil and dust, which has accumulated and bound lead over the decades from airborne pollution.

Many years ago, I have a 2 years old patient referred to me with a lead level of over 10. While talking to mom, we discovered that the child had been eating his meals and snack off of the antique lacquer furnitures in the house. The child would touch and play on the furnitures, and eat his meals/snacks on the furnitures as well.

Other sources of exposure include water (leaching from lead in pipes, as in the recent Flint water crisis) and lead in imported toys, jewelry, candles, canned foods, candy wrappers, cosmetics, and poorly regulated dietary supplements.

Children who live near airports are exposed to air polluted with leaded jet fuel from airplanes.

If your child has ADHD, consider checking your environment for possible lead sources as listed above and making corrections as much as possible.

2. Mercury

Mercury is a neurotoxin, exposure to which is linked to brain and nervous system damage, kidney damage, autoimmune, and other health effects.

Separate research had also revealed that babies exposed in the womb to higher levels of mercury, due to their mom's fish-rich diet, scored lower on skill tests when they became infants and toddlers.

A study showed children exposed to higher levels of mercury in the womb are more likely to show attention problems, hyperactivity, and other ADHD symptoms when they're 8 years old.

Researchers measured the mercury levels in the mothers' hair shortly after birth and found that a child's risk of ADHD symptoms increased by 40% to 70% past a certain exposure threshold (1 microgram per gram).

The health effects of mercury toxicity depend on a variety of factors, including the form and amount of mercury and the developmental age of the person being exposed.

The majority of mercury exposure comes from eating fish from mercury-contaminated waters. This is why the U.S. Food and Drug Administration recommends that pregnant women consume no more than two six-ounce servings of low-mercury fish per week.

Smaller, oily fishes such as salmon, herring, mackerel, and sardines tend to be low in mercury and yet high in omega-3s, which is beneficial for preventing ADHD in an unborn child.

Shark, swordfish, and fresh tuna, on the other hand, contain high levels of mercury and a relatively modest amount of omega-3s. Therefore, these fish should be avoided.

Mercury in Your Mouth?

Yes…in fact, each time you eat, drink, brush your teeth or otherwise stimulate your teeth.

There is overwhelming evidence that shows mercury vapor being released from dental fillings each time you eat, drink, brush your teeth, or otherwise stimulate your teeth.

This mercury vapor readily enters your cell membranes, across your blood-brain barrier into your central nervous system and can cause all kinds of psychological, neurological, and immunological problems.

Dental amalgam filling, aka "silver fillings," has no silver at all. It contains more mercury than any other product sold in the United States. They are cheap and easy to install compared to mercury-free composite fillings. That's why they're the first choice in any dentist's office, and their profit margins are high.

Mercury found in contaminated fish, and dental amalgam is methyl mercury, the type that is readily absorbed by the body and accumulates.

"Thimerosal" is mercury found in vaccines, which is made of ethyl mercury. Ethyl mercury is less likely to accumulate or cause ill effects compared to methyl mercury because it is eliminated from the body much more quickly.

Mercury is also found in many common everyday products, such as batteries, thermometers and barometers, electric switches and relays in equipment, lamps (including some types of light bulbs), skin-lightening products and other cosmetics.

3. Organophosphate Pesticides

Organophosphate insecticides are one of the most commonly used pesticides worldwide. You'll find it in just about anywhere, such as homes, veterinary offices, and farms.

Organophosphate interferes with the acetylcholinesterase enzyme (AChE), causing too much acetylcholine (ACh) to accumulate. This results in behavioral changes, respiratory issues, and coordination problems when it affects the central nervous system (CNS).

Most people get exposed to organophosphates by consuming contaminated food and water. Children are at much higher risk for organophosphate toxicity because the developing brain is more susceptible to neurotoxins than mature adult brains. The dose of pesticides per body weight is likely to be more significant for children.

Organophosphate exposure in children has been linked to multiple problems, though the type varies depending on the time of exposure.

It is also known that exposure to organophosphate during pregnancy was associated with an increased risk of pervasive developmental disorders and delays in mental development.

Exposure to organophosphate after birth has been associated with behavioral problems, such as poorer short-term memory and motor skills, and slow reaction times in children.

It is well known that certain commercially produced fruits and vegetables are loaded with significant organophosphates and should be avoided.

Each year the *Environmental Work Group* publishes a list of produce to avoid and buy organic only called "*The Dirty Dozen.*"

See the "Brain Kryptonite Food to Avoid" in the Appendix for the full Dirty Dozen to avoid.

4. Prenatal Tobacco Exposure

Prenatal nicotine exposure increases the risk for children developing ADHD later in life. Higher levels of nicotine were associated with a greater risk for ADHD, and the association between smoking and ADHD has a dose-response effect.

Children born to women who smoke cigarettes during pregnancy, especially when mothers are heavy smokers, are at an increased risk for ADHD. Mothers who smoked during pregnancy had an overall 60 percent higher risk of having a child with ADHD compared to women who didn't smoke.

Seven studies showed that while mothers' smoking had a more significant effect than fathers' smoking on ADHD risk, there was still a 20 percent higher risk of ADHD in children born to fathers who smoked.

5. Bisphenol A or BPA

Bisphenols A or BPA is another dangerous food additive for ADHD that disrupts hormonal systems. BPA, a petrochemical derivative used to stiffen plastics, but it acts like estrogen in the body.

BPAs can act like the hormone estrogen and interfere with puberty, fertility, and increase the risk of hormone-related cancers.

Bisphenols can also increase body fat and cause problems with the immune system and nervous system resulting in behavioral and metabolic disorders.

According to a study published in the journal Environmental Research, children with high levels of the chemical bisphenol-A in their bodies were more likely to have ADHD than those with lower levels.

Bisphenols are found in the *lining of food and soda cans* to prevent the metal from eroding. They're also found in plastic containers labeled with *numbers 3 or 7*.

Can you imagine these used to be in plastic baby bottles and sippy cups too? Fortunately, that's history. BPAs now are banned, but older bottles and containers may still contain them.

EWG published a report that reveals more than 16,000 processed foods may be packaged in materials that contain BPA. People can also be exposed to BPA through thermal cashier receipts. So ask for your receipt to be emailed.

6. Electronic Media Exposure

Working in the pediatric clinic, I see kids as young as one-year-old using an electronic device. We always joke about how parents use the iPad or tablet as a babysitter.

Two studies looked at the association between television and video game exposure and ADHD.

The Japanese study found that children with high levels of television viewing at 18 months of age had greater hyperactive and inattention symptoms at 30 months of age compared with those with low exposure.

The other study looked at the association between hours of television and video game use and attention problems in both school-aged children and young adults, and found an association between higher total screen time (television plus video games) and increased attention problems.

7. Artificial Food Additives

One day I picked up my daughter from after school care as usual. She was unusually energetic and talkative that day. Usually, she'd just get into the car asked about what's for dinner. She might tell me a few things that happened in school that day.

But this day was different. It's almost like her motor was on high gear. She talked at way higher speed than her usual with extra energy level, which I had never seen in her before.

If you read my story, you know my daughter had a speech delay, so talking is not her thing.

This happens a few more times, and I finally figured that it's the pepperoni she ate at the after school care.

After that, no more pepperoni or deli meats for her, or anything with food additives.

Reactions to chemicals in food, such as preservatives, monosodium glutamate, red food dye, high fructose corn syrup, and the other thousands of food additives in our food system, can manifest as anger, agitation, impulsivity, hyperactivity and lack of concentration.

This is the basis of the Feingold diet, discovered by Dr. Benjamin Feingold in 1975.

Dr. Feingold discovered that when he removed certain food additives, such as food colorings, preservatives, salicylates, etc., many of his patients' hyperactive behaviors also improved along with their allergic reactions.

He noticed *improvements in hyperactivity, impulsivity, compulsive actions, attention span, cognitive and perceptual disturbances, along with improvements in skin problems/hives, and sleep problems.*

Did I mention that Dr. Feingold was an allergist?

He was not a psychiatrist. He made this discovery by accident when he was treating his patients for food sensitivities.

1. Artificial Food Coloring

Chances are if you buy any processed food, you'll come across artificial food coloring. The only exception is shopping from Whole Foods, Trader Joe's, or Thrive Market.

I used to love Cheetos and Doritos. Can you imagine how much food coloring, preservatives, and other chemicals are in these "junk food"?

Artificial food coloring is one of the worst food additives for ADHD. Many of these artificial food colorings are banned in European countries after a British study linked them to hyperactivity in children.

Studies show that artificial food colorings may contribute to asthma and hyperactivity in children and may also lead to a significant reduction in intelligent quotient (I.Q.).

Studies have also linked artificial food colorings to thyroid cancer, kidney and adrenal gland tumors, and DNA gene damage in laboratory animals that may also interfere with brain chemistry.

2. Preservatives

Butylated hydroxyanisole (BHA), butylated hydroxytoluene (BHT), and TBHQ (Tertiary Butylhydroquinone) are preservatives used to extend the shelf-life of fatty foods. These preservatives prevent foods from changing color, changing the flavor, or becoming rancid.

While the food is looking pretty with these preservatives, your brain is not so when you ingest them.

These preservatives are shown to *affects the brain and behavior and increase the risk of cancer.*

You'll find them in just about anything from potato chips, nuts, nut butter, salad dressing, instant noodles, canned meats, and vegetable oils.

3. Artificial Sweeteners

If you're like most people who think "diet drinks" are better and drink these over regular soda or juice, think again.

I generally advise all my families to avoid artificial sweeteners because the studies that confirmed their safety are all paid for by the manufacturers. Second, most of the reviews are done on adults.

Who in the right mind would want their child to be a guinea pig?

That means, no one knows how these man-made artificial sweeteners would affect growth in young children, who is still growing and developing rapidly.

Now newer studies are coming out showing the actual effects of these so-called "healthy sugar alternatives" or "it's natural because it's made from sugar".

Well…cyanide is natural too. Does that mean it's right for you?

Aspartame (Nutrasweet and Equal) is toxic to the brain and can cause cancer. It affects intelligence and short-term memory. This toxic sweetener may be linked to diseases like lymphoma, diabetes, multiple sclerosis, Parkinson's, Alzheimer's, fibromyalgia, and chronic fatigue, emotional disorders like depression and anxiety attacks, dizziness, headaches, nausea, mental confusion, migraines and seizures, and possibly brain masses.

You'll find this sweetener in manufactured baked goods, chewing gum, gelatin, diet soda, and flavored water.

Sucralose (Splenda) can cause damages to your liver, kidneys, and thymus gland. Sucralose pretends to be natural with claims that "it is made from sugar." The chemical structure of sucralose looks more like sugar.

Results from several large population studies suggest regular use of artificial sweeteners like aspartame and sucralose increase insulin resistance and increase risks of weight gain and diabetes.

Acesulfame potassium is usually used with other artificial sweeteners in diet sodas and sugar-free dessert. It is linked to cancer of the lungs and breasts and possibly kidney as well.

Saccharin (Sweet n Low) is a cancer-causing substance found to cause bladder cancer in lab rats studies.

Artificial sweeteners can be found in just about every processed item, even toothpaste. But for sure anything that says "*diet*" *or* "*sugar-free*".

4. High Fructose Corn Syrup

Sugar is bad. We all know that. But how bad is sugar for kids with ADHD?

Parents often report their children became crazy hyper after eating loads of sugar or refined carb. Is that just a coincidence, or does sugar make your child hyper?

According to a study in the Journal of Nutrition, a high intake of sweets and processed carbohydrates are associated with four times more risks of ADHD...FOUR TIMES!

Sugar intake over the last 40 years has increased thanks to the introduction of high fructose corn syrup significantly. Today, "added sugar" (not the same as natural sugar) accounts for 15-20% of adult daily intake.

Unlike the artificial sweeteners we read about earlier, high fructose corn syrup is used to significantly enhance the food's flavors to an almost addicting level.

Yes, to an addicting level. If you think you or your child are addicted to sugar or sweets, chances are "yes, you're addicted to sugar".

What are the symptoms of sugar addiction?

Same as heroin and cocaine addiction...seriously.

High fructose corn syrup (HFCS) is a *highly-processed artificial sweetener*, which has become the number one source of excess calories in America. It is found in almost every processed food.

This empty-calorie substance not only provides the *extra bursts of energy in children with ADHD*, but it also *interferes with your child's brain neurotransmitters and chemistry*.

It interferes with the dopamine reward system. With long-term use, it exhausts the dopamine reward system, causing an addictive effect similar to addictive behaviors seen in cocaine and heroin users.

When you eat food with sugar and HFCS, it stimulates your brain to make dopamine (the feel food signal). That's why sweets always make you happy.

As you eat more food that contains sugar and HFCS, your brain continues to make more dopamine. However, over time, your brain needs to make more and more dopamine to get the same "sugar high", eventually the dopamine receptors in the brain get worn out and not responding to dopamine anymore.

When you eat yummy food, your brain makes dopamine too due to the novelty of the food. But this dopamine response slows down as you eat more of this new delicious food.

But when human overeats sugar, dopamine release continues similar overtime despite higher sugar intake, which suggests "desensitization".

Studies in rats show that rats who's become so addicted to sugar that they'd ignore the painful "foot shock" to get to the sugar.

Not all sugar is addicting. Table sugar or sucrose breaks up into a molecule of glucose and a molecule of fructose.

Glucose is the good sugar because it can be used by all our cells for energy and is essential for some parts of our bodies. The best sources of natural carbohydrates are starchy vegetables. Glucose does not have the same addicting effects as fructose.

Fructose can only be metabolized by the liver and can't be used for energy by your body's cells. It's not only entirely useless for the body, but it's also toxic in high amounts because the liver has to get rid of it, mainly by turning it into fat and storing it in the liver. Eventually, fatty liver happens.

Fructose also causes obesity by blocking leptin secretion, induce insulin, and leptin resistance. Fructose also depletes ATP, energy in the liver and hypothalamus, increasing sense of hunger.

Do you know who else loves sugar too? Bacteria, and yeast. For you pastry and bread maker out there, you know very well how to make the best bread dough. You feed the yeast with sugar first, so the bread dough rises nicely.

While most of your body's cells can't use fructose as a source of energy, the bacteria in your gut can and too much fructose can create gut flora imbalances, promote bacterial overgrowth and promote the growth of pathogenic bacteria.

Sugar causes obesity, which is common in kids with ADHD. When you eat carbs or sugar, your body responds with insulin to direct the sugar into tissue cells for energy. However, when you eat highly processed refined carbohydrates, there's a sudden rush of blood sugar, your body panic, and make excess insulin to direct the blood sugar into tissue cells quickly.

Now two things bad is happening here:

- Too much sugar going into tissue cells faster than the cells can use, the extra sugar is turned into fat for storage.

- High insulin level blocks the body from using fat as back up energy source. The insulin rush causes the blood sugar to tank, at the same time, you can't tap into the backup fat energy, you're starving and cranky. Cravings happen.

This cravings plus the addicting effects of sugar make it almost impossible to say no to sugar. Then you repeat the whole process the binging eating sugar all day long.

This is the horror story of ADHD and obesity. Twenty-three percent of ADHD kids are obese and have binge eating disorder due poor self-control with deficiency in norepinephrine.

Kids who are used to the sweetness of high fructose corn syrup have difficulty accepting the more natural sweetness of real fruits. A good rule of thumb is to limit fructose to less than **20 grams per day**. Keeping in mind that **most fruits are half glucose and half fructose**, so eating too many fruits can become problematic.

5. Monosodium Glutamate or MSG

You've heard of "Chinese restaurant syndrome", which is an outdated term coined in the 1960s. It refers to a group of symptoms some people experience after eating a Chinese restaurant, which is often the additive monosodium glutamate (MSG). These symptoms often include headaches, skin flushing, and sweating. Today, it's known as "MSG Symptom Complex".

MSG is another dangerous food additive for children with ADHD. It is toxic to the brain and may cause brain cells to die. It is associated with worsening learning disabilities, ADHD, Alzheimer's disease, Parkinson's disease, Lou Gehrig's disease, and more.

Studies show that eating food with MSG frequently may result in depression, disorientation, eye damage, fatigue, headaches, and obesity.

Yes, MSG is also the ingredient that makes you want to eat more, and pack on the weight.

If you or your child has ADHD, you should definitely avoid these dangerous food additives that may trigger your ADHD symptoms by interfering with normal brain chemistry.

It is commonly used in food prepared in many Asian restaurants. It is also used to enhance flavors in soups, salad dressings, chips, frozen entrees, and lunch meats.

Can your child's delicate growing body handle all these poisons in our food supply?

Every Child is Different

My job is to care for children with special needs and other rare genetic disorders, so I understand every one of our own uniqueness at a molecular and genetic level.

It is the same reason why ten breast cancer patients with the same treatment will have ten different outcomes.

Conventional medicine is guessing most of the time, as much as everyone else is here.

Conventional medicine practices "evidence-based medicine," which basically means, "we'll going to use the treatment with the most positive response from studies. These studies show this particular treatment works 70% of the time, which is more than half, so it should work for you too. What's your name now?"

They don't even look at who you are but treating you as a diagnosis. "You have ADHD. Take this medicine."

We all need to remember that each of us is genetically different in some minor ways; that is, each of us interprets taste and smell differently and reacts to food and chemical differently.

Therefore, it makes sense that some children may be more sensitive to certain food additives, food coloring, and preservatives used in processed food. Some of us just have a harder time dealing with environmental toxins in our environment and suffer more environmental allergies.

This also explains why your friend's child did well with a particular supplement, which does nothing for your child, or it made your child's symptoms worse.

However, every human being needs the same basic nutrients - amino acids, fatty acids, glucose, vitamins, minerals, and antioxidants to survive and thrive. There's no doubt about that unless you're an alien.

Nutrition Comes First

Studies have found a strong connection between food and nutrition intake, digestion, and ADHD symptoms. This is the reason why when parents told their pediatricians that they don't want to start their child on ADHD medications, they send these families to me for dietary changes.

Studies compared a standard American diet to a special elimination diet and found that the special elimination diet resulted in a dramatic reduction in ADHD symptoms.

In my practice with children with ADHD, I have seen many patients reduce or even resolved their ADHD symptoms by simply improving the quality of their child's diet.

Many parents are completely unaware that their child has a food sensitivity, especially if the food that bothers them is something they eat every day or are considered healthy, like wheat and dairy products.

A few years ago, a 5-year-old girl was referred to me for being too skinny because she's a picky eater and refuses to drink cow's milk.

After some questioning about the picky eater, diet history, and review of all symptoms, I told the mom that her child is picky and refuses milk because she has a cow's milk allergy since she was a baby.

She has all the classic signs and symptoms of cow's milk protein allergy since birth - projectile vomiting, constipation, blood in the stool, eczema. The problem was not caught and just ditched her symptoms as something "she will outgrow it."

I usually diagnosed children with cow's milk protein allergy during the first year of age. And this girl is five years old. I told the mom that it might take her a lot longer to outgrow the milk allergy if she ever would, as she's been continually exposed to cow's milk all her life.

Heavy advertising by the dairy industry brainwashed every pediatrician and parent to force milk to their kids every day, even to the point of ignoring the symptoms after drinking milk.

I was guilty of that too until I realized my daughter was reacting to cow's milk when she had too much of it.

Every child is different, so one food that is bothersome for one child may not bother another child at all.

Unfortunately, not all foods are equal. Some food nourishes the brain, while others deplete the brain. So what do you want the food your child eats every day to do?

Eating the right kinds of food and nutrition will give your child's ADHD brain the boost it needs to stay focused, energized, and happy all day long.

Imagine you just bought this beautiful home and you want to do some renovations and upgrades because some of the appliances look old.

Sound awesome, right?

But there's a problem. There's no electricity. How do you know which piece of appliance works and which one not?

Proper nutrition is the electricity that powers your child's body and brain functions.

Even though electricity is an analogy here, the brain does communicate in electricity or electrical impulses.

So nutrition therapy should come first before any other treatment. We need to get the electricity to the brain so we can turn on the light to see what's going on.

The ADHD symptoms and behaviors are only telling us something is not working right in the brain connection, but we don't know what exactly it is until we turn on the electricity.

It's easy to assume that your child's lethargy, disengaged demeanor, and tantrums are entirely due to his ADHD diagnosis until you see all of these behaviors improve with proper nutrition interventions.

Watching a child's attitude and ability to change when he is fully nourished is always an eye-opener.

Using nutrition therapy for a child with special needs can be complicated. Parents need support, guidance, expertise, resources, and encouragement for it. This book is meant to help you through this journey.

Nutrition therapy can be a very potent natural ADHD treatment that can work very well if done correctly. We need to give the brain the fundamental basics - a clean nourishing diet free of trigger foods, toxic food additives, and processed sugar and starches.

Feeding your child proper nutrition doesn't just put a band-aid on the ADHD symptoms as conventional ADHD medications do, it fixes the problem at the root cause level.

From that perspective, I've found that dietary strategies as the cornerstone of a successful natural ADHD remedy program.

Remember, ADHD does not doom your child to a life of under-achievement and failure. Many of the world's most significant discoveries and inventions were made by people with ADHD.

If you're ready, let's get started…

EAT TO FOCUS Natural ADHD Treatment Protocol

In this chapter, you'll learn more about each of the 4 phases that will transform your child's ADHD symptoms and your family life.

I know there's an ADHD diet that works and it's not as simple as your usual "healthy" diet.

Remember *when you're pregnant, you watch what you eat* and make sure your child gets the best start in life?

When *your baby was born, you try your best to feed your baby the best food you can*.

Brand-new parents would do anything they can to make sure that only the best nutrition goes into their kids' bodies.

E*very parent knows how important nutrition is for their children's health*. So it seems *as a society we agree that food and nutrition are essential*.

We are what we eat is true.

Touch your nose with your finger. Do you feel your nose? Where does your nose come from that you can feel and touch? Where does the nerve that helps you move your arm to your nose come from?

Everything on your body comes from the food you put in your body from the time you're conceived.

If you change your child's diet in a good way and you notice improvements in his or her behaviors, then who cares what the studies said. The most important thing is it works for your child.

After working in the healthcare field for over 19 years, scientific studies and researches are great but only prove, at their best, what is most likely to happen to a specific population. Just because 70% of the studied population responds to a particular treatment does not mean the other 30% possibility does not exists.

We need to stay open-minded. We all need to remember each of us is genetically different in our unique ways, like a snowflake.

The diet of the many kids I see with ADHD consists mostly of processed packaged food with minimal real food. Their only fruit source is fruit cups or fruit snacks. And their vegetables are mainly French fries, ketchup and corn.

Over the years, I've not had a parent who told me that improving their child's diet does not work. It always works. The question is to what extend.

Let's start with the "*Healthy Diet Dilemma*."

It's the healthy diet that everyone talks about and follow, shouldn't it be good for ADHD?

From magazine ads to TV commercials to your doctors, families, and friends, and other nutritionists, they all tell you "eat low calories, eat low-fat, eat low cholesterol, eat low salt, eat sugar-free food, eat whole grains, eat whole wheat, drink your milk" and so on, and on…

I'm going to bust all of these and explain why the conventional "healthy diet" is harmful to kids with ADHD.

1. A "healthy diet" is *excessive in the wrong carbs*. People everywhere eating *beans, whole wheat, and whole grain, thinking that these are the magical healthy foods*. I'm sorry to burst your bubbles. But granola, brown rice, whole-wheat pasta, whole wheat bread, and beans we eat today are *highly modified genetically*. Meaning our human body cannot recognize and process these grains. Kids with ADHD do not handle carbs well. And remember, we talked about gluten sensitivity in kids with ADHD. People with ADHD are also more likely to have Celiac disease. Fifteen percent of people with ADHD have Celiac disease, compared to only 1% in the general population.

2. Fats are friends not foes. Fat matters even more so to your child than you think. Kids need fats to build new brain and organ tissues. Your body can only get fat-soluble vitamins A, D, E, K from fats only. A low-fat diet is deficient in fat-soluble vitamins and energy. Dietary cholesterol is not the cause of high blood cholesterol or the origins of cardiovascular diseases. The 300mg cholesterol daily limit is a fraud, is supported by no studies. Your body makes 85% of the cholesterol in your blood. The question you should be asking is, why is your body making so much cholesterol? By the way, children need cholesterol in their diet because cholesterol is necessary to stabilize the cell membrane. If the cell membrane is unstable, the cell cannot function properly, and bad things happen.

3. Sugar-free and diet food and beverages are poisonous. The studies that showed artificial sugar is safe are *studies paid for by the manufacturers of these artificial sweeteners*. The sugar has no calories because the *body cannot recognize it and cannot use it*. Recent new studies show that these sugar-free foods or artificial sweeteners still *stimulate the same reward receptor in the brain (aka the dopamine center), just like real sugar, which means they even trigger sugar cravings in the brain*. Scientists also show that these artificial sugar *increase risk of insulin resistance and obesity*. In ADHD, this means the brain has an even harder time to use sugar and carbs from the diet.

The "healthy diet" is not so healthy, after all.

In the previous chapters, we learned about the five underlying causes of ADHD.

1. We learn that *the ADHD brain is smaller and behind other children's minds by an average of 3 years*. And it *does not process carbs and sugar well*. It also has low brain chemical levels.

Diet strategies: high-fat food boosts brain catch-up growth, low sugar & stable carbs to avoid sugar cravings, and high protein food to support brain chemical production.

2. We also learn that the *ADHD brain communicates with the gut constantly, and when the gut is imbalanced, it feeds the ADHD brain the wrong signals.* And we also learn that the imbalanced gut is caused by yeast and or bacterial overgrowth.

Diet strategies: low sugar to starve off yeast and harmful bacteria, high fiber food to feed the good bacteria, probiotics food or supplements to bring in more good bacteria, digestive enzymes to improve digestion, and collagen protein to heal the leaky gut.

3. We then learn that *kids with ADHD have many hidden food intolerances that over-stimulate the immune system causing unnecessary inflammation that results in the many forms of ADHD symptoms*.

Diet strategies: elimination diet that eliminates common food allergens, dairy, soy, grains, corn, peanuts, beans, eggs, and nuts to identify trouble foods.

4. We also learn about the *four most common nutrient deficiencies in kids with ADHD* - omega-3 fatty acids, magnesium, zinc, and iron.

Diet strategies include natural minerals from organic fruits and vegetables, healthy fats, unrefined sea salts, and supplements with fish oil, magnesium, zinc, and iron.

5. And we learn that environmental toxins in our food and environment can affect brain chemistry and the body's hormonal systems, causing ADHD symptoms.

Diet strategies: choose organic, non-GMO animal products, and produce. Avoid processed mass-produced food that contains artificial synthetic food additives.

Does this make sense?

Based on what we know so far about the possible causes of ADHD, the best ADHD diet that works for your child needs to:

- *improve digestion*

- *correct nutrient deficiencies*
- *promote body's own detoxification*
- *calm the over-reacting immune system*
- *reduce systemic inflammation*

This may seem like a lot to do. That's why I created this simple and easy four-step protocol so that you can take it one step at a time.

The *Eat to Focus Protocol* is your roadmap of the functional approach to reducing hyperactivity and impulsivity without drug side effects.

The objectives of the **Eat to Focus Protocol** is to:

1. Reduce hyperactivity and impulsivity
2. Improve focus and memory
3. Minimize anger outburst and mood meltdowns
4. Improve grades and school work
5. Improve social relationships with friends and family

The **Eat to Focus Protocol** will help you identify the underlying causes of your child's ADHD symptoms and design your own natural treatment program to getting your child to reduce hyperactivity, impulsiveness and anxiety, and improve focus and memory.

The goal is to support and nourish your child's whole body from the inside out.

Here are the four simple steps to help you get started:

1. **Clean Start.** This is the elimination phase of the program. You remove brain-whacking foods and toxins to relieve the toxic burden on the body and brain.
    - Avoid common food triggers, such as dairy, soy, grains, beans, peanut, corn, eggs, and nuts.
    - Avoid processed foods, foods that come out from a package or box, frozen meals, frozen dinner, fast foods, cereal, cookies, chips, crackers, candies, granola, fruit juices, fruit snacks, soda or pop, sugary snacks, table sugar, syrup, and artificial sugar.
    - Avoid GMOs as much as possible. I know 100% is not possible. But try your best.

2. Feed the ADHD Brain. Now we know the ADHD brain functions slightly different than normal developing child's brain. In this step, you focus on clean nutrient-rich brain foods to boost catch-up brain growth and fuel the ADHD brain properly along with supplements to correct nutrient deficiencies.
- organic animal protein, low glycemic index fruits, and vegetables
- healthy fats from non-GMO sources
- unrefined sea salts

- supplements to correct common nutrient deficiencies

3. Feed the ADHD Gut. We learned about the strong connection between the brain functions and gut functions; and that the gut makes most of the brain chemicals in our body. Therefore, fixing the gut will help improve many of the explosive behaviors.
- avoid sugar
- eat high fiber slow carb fruits and vegetables
- eat organ meat and bone broth for collagen (or supplements),
- eat fermented foods and beverages, probiotics supplements
- take digestive enzymes

4. Brain Reboot. The previous three steps focus on optimizing brain functions, and growth. This final step focuses on brain development with scientifically proven activities to support creating new brain connections.

This step is kind of like having an architect to direct the building of your new home, so you don't end up with a toilet in the kitchen.

Well, that's an extreme example.

But you get my point, right?

Connections between brain cells get stronger the more often it is repeated (or practiced), the so-called muscle memory. And muscle memory is not only for the muscle. It's in the brain too.

We'll talk about topics on:

- sleep hygiene
- physical activities
- mindfulness

As your child progresses through the steps, your child's hyperactivity, impulsivity, attention, mood, and sleep will start to improve to the point that you may skip the "Healing Hours."

But I still recommend that you go through all the steps to understand why your child is behaving the way he or she is.

Why Follow The Eat to Focus Protocol?

This is the only program out there that shows you step-by-step of all the things you need to help your child stay calm and focus without medication.

Other programs either just want to sell you some supplements that either do not work or work only for a little while. Or some shows you the conventional "healthy diet "that does more harm than good.

None of these other programs take into deeper consideration the multifactorial aspects of ADHD.

You cannot expect your child ADHD symptoms just magically improve just taking a supplement pill, or simply eating more protein at breakfast or removing food coloring or salicylates.

People frequently fail to realize that the many underlying causes of ADHD have a lot to do with what you put into your body.

The ***Eat to Focus Protocol*** is the ultimate lifestyle protocol that helps children and adults with ADHD overcome the core underlying causes of ADHD symptoms and behavioral disorders. These include systemic inflammation, leaky gut, blood sugar imbalances, nutrient deficiencies, and an over-reactive immune system.

Our goal is not to just put a bandaid on the symptoms. Our goal is symptom resolution.

The most important thing to realize is that you have the power to change right now.

The *Eat to Focus Protocol* is a therapeutic protocol that eliminates environmental toxins, including foods and additives known to trigger immune and systemic inflammation that cause ADHD behaviors and symptoms, while rebuilding damaged gut lining and creating new nerve connections.

1. **Support Gut Health**: The gut is our first line of defense against all incoming invaders, namely nasty bacteria and critters. If the gut function is compromised, it means digestion is affecting, meaning food is not being digested and absorbed properly. Then it does not matter if you're eating organic grass-fed bison hand-fed and massaged daily by Prince Henry. The food will just rot and ferment in the intestine, causing inflammation, gut dysbiosis (imbalances in gut bacteria), and a leaky gut. Then more undigested food particles can enter the bloodstream causing an unnecessary immune response. The first phase of the *Eat to Focus* focuses on eliminating foods that irritate the gut lining.

2. **Regulate Immune System**: Seventy-five percent of our body's immunity is in the GI tract. Inflammation, leaky gut, hormone imbalance, blood sugar imbalances, and micronutrient deficiencies contribute to an overactive immune system. By rebalancing the gut bacteria, reducing inflammation in the gut, removing food triggers from your diet, and supporting blood sugar regulation, the *Eat to Focus* protocol helps to improve immune function.

3. Eliminate Chronic Inflammation: Processed food, artificial food additives, and certain trigger foods can damage intestines lining and contribute to low-grade systemic inflammation and autoimmune response that are responsible for some of the ADHD symptoms and behaviors. Foods that irritate the bowel and cause leaky gut are avoided.

4. Balance Blood Sugar: Fluctuating blood sugar can not only causes mood swings, but also lead to systemic inflammation, immune flares, and compromised brain function. Therefore, balancing blood sugar levels is essential to keep inflammatory at bay. The *Eat to Focus* protocol gives you the tools and resources to support healthy balanced blood sugar and moods while reducing inflammation.

5. Support Brain Growth & Development: Children are growing every second of the day, you don't want to take that away from them. Every cell in the body is kept alive by thousands of biochemical reactions powered by a vitamin, a mineral, an antioxidant, or a combination of them. Feeding the body with foods loaded with essential vitamins, minerals, and antioxidants guarantees the body and all systems function in top shape to support healthy growth and learning. And this starts with the right diet.

How to Use The *Eat to Focus* Protocol?

The *Eat to Focus Protocol* consists of four phases - **Clean Start, Feed the ADHD Brain, Feed the ADHD Gut,** and **Brain Reboot**.

For eight weeks or longer, you eliminate all foods that are known to potentially trigger allergic reactions and inflammation that result in ADHD symptoms.

Following at least eight weeks of elimination with most symptoms disappeared, you may re-introduce one food back at a time to see if your body is well enough to tolerate these foods again.

If you re-introduce a food back, and symptoms return, then you'll know that food should be avoided. On the other hand, if you re-introduce a food, and no symptoms return, then that food is good and you can continue to eat it.

In my practice, I usually have my patients re-introduce food that they used to eat the most frequently or missed the most.

The optimal end result is a diet and lifestyle that support your child's mental and emotional health without triggering systemic inflammation and unnecessary immune reaction.

PHASE 1

CLEAN START

"We are what we eat...therefore...garbage in and garbage out."

The use of an elimination diet for neurological disorders, including ADHD is not new. The idea of elimination diet to treat neurological disorders had been around since the 1920's.

Reports of adverse physical reactions to foods (eg, eczema, asthma, and gastrointestinal problems) have led to the suggestion that foods might also affect the brain, resulting in adverse behavioral effects.

A ketogenic diet, which eliminates almost all carbohydrates from the diet, has been used for seizure control by Dr. Russell Wilder at the Mayo Clinic since the 1923.

In 1975, Dr. Benjamin Feingold, a pediatric allergist, discovered that eliminating artificial food coloring, flavorings, salicylates, etc. reduced hyperactivity and impulsivity in children.

In 1989, Egger studied 45 epileptic children. Twenty-five stopped having seizures and eleven had significantly fewer seizures during an elimination diet therapy.

In 2001, Frediani *et al.* also looked at 72 epileptic children and 202 healthy control, age-matched individuals with their families. They found higher incidence of cow's milk allergy and asthma in epileptic children group, and dermatitis and rhinitis in their mothers and their siblings, respectively.

Benefits of Elimination Diet & ADHD

Many many years ago, when I first started looking into natural alternative ADHD treatment, everything that I read says there's no conclusive evidence to show dietary intervention works.

But at the same time, I was hearing all these success stories from families, especially families of children with autism. If autism can be treated successfully with dietary changes, then diet must work.

As the years go by, more and more studies and research come out to support the effects of diet composition on kids and their behaviors.

Many studies show that diet composition and meal patterns can have immediate and long-term effects on children's full genetic potential. These factors can affect their physical growth and mental development.

And it's been proven that dietary changes can improve brain functions and behaviors in children and adolescents, who have poor nutritional status. Scientists also showed that elimination diets could help kids with ADHD improve their symptoms.

A growing number of researches suggests that diets that eliminate both toxic additives and potential allergens, while loaded with nutrient-rich foods, may play a significant role in the management of ADHD.

A review in 2004 looked at 15 double-blind, placebo-controlled (these are the king of studies) studies. The review concluded that *there was a positive effect linking synthetic food colorings to ADHD symptoms*. These studies focused on food coloring elimination.

Another widely publicized population-based study conducted in England concluded that food additives contribute to hyperactivity. The result of this study prompts the European Union Parliament to take action immediately.

In Europe, warning labels are now required to identify food that contains artificial food coloring.

In 2011, a double-blind crossover study of an elimination diet randomized 50 children with ADHD to an individually designed elimination diet and 50 to just "healthy diet" counseling. Thirty children (60%) respond positively to the "individualized" elimination diet, and only 19 of the 30 had symptom relapse when the trigger food were re-introduced.

Processed fast food and beverages are like **Trojan horses.** You eat things that look like food, but you're putting a bunch of harmful critters into your body that hijacks your child's command center (brain).

A diet consists mainly of processed foods robs your body of the precious vitamins and minerals your body craves. Still, it also fills your body with toxic chemicals, pesticides, hormones, and preservatives, which affect the body's hormone system and cause unnecessary inflammation.

Your body ends up using most of its resources to get rid of these junks and try to recover while trying to grow and learn in the case of a young child.

If your current diet consists of many processed and packaged food, fast food, etc., some of your symptoms may disappear after removing majority of foods that contain artificial food additives.

What is Clean Start?

Clean Start helps you remove *specific ingredients, additives, and foods from the diet to reduce ADHD symptoms caused by such foods*.

These are *usually foods suspected of causing allergic or autoimmune reactions* or food that contains synthetic food additives.

Clean Start is *very effective in identifying and treating food allergy and sensitivity.*

You can have an *allergic response to food.* Symptoms of reactions include itchy skin, sensitivity/swelling in the mouth, rhinitis, breathing difficulties, and gastrointestinal issues ranging from vomiting, constipation, diarrhea, blood in the stool, and less well-known nervous symptoms, like headache, anxiety, confusion, nervousness, and tiredness.

On the other hand, food intolerance is a nonallergic response to a food item, which may be due to enzyme deficiency (e.g., lactose intolerance) or another non-immunological hypersensitivity reaction such as to food additives.

Food intolerance can also cause digestive problems, but too often result in other non-specific symptoms, such as headaches, blurred vision, mood changes, fatigue, and aches and pains.

ADHD symptoms can also involve food hypersensitivity or intolerance to chemicals found in food, such as salicylates.

When you nourish your body with the right food and nutrition the way God made them, you'll nourish your body, mind, and soul.

This is the reason why *Clean Start* is the first phase.

How Do You Know If Your Child Have Hidden Food Sensitivity?

When people think of food allergies, they're thinking of an immediate physical reaction just like the scene of Will Smith in the movie *HITCH*, where he accidentally ate something with shrimp which he is severely allergic to. He immediately started having problem with breathing, itchy skin, and facial swellings.

But the allergies or food intolerance that I'm talking about or commonly seen in children with ADHD are a lot more subtle than that.

Most kids with ADHD suffer from what we called delayed food reaction or what sometimes call "hidden food allergies" or food intolerances.

These reactions to food showed up hours, sometimes up to days after eating certain food.

It took me years to figure out that I have a gluten sensitivity because I don't feel anything until about 3 days after eating gluten containing foods.

In kids, sometimes the only symptoms you have is just "picky eater, who refused to eat most food and have no interest in eating because young children does not have the verbal skills to voice their discomfort.

Maybe you have food allergy testing done for your child, and all the tests come back negative...I hear you.

I had food allergy testing done, both the RAST and skin prick, and all were negative. But I know I'm not crazy and making up symptoms in my head. I have asthma, and I know something triggers it.

I also have sensitivities to gluten and wheat products and other foods, but nothing shows up on the allergy tests.

The truth of the matter is hidden allergies are not detected in the RAST or skin prick tests, which are looking for IgE-mediated reactions.

Food allergy that causes neurological symptoms are not IgE-mediated, but mostly IgG-mediated. And symptoms usually appeared on average 2-3 days after ingestion of trigger foods, which make these food allergies super difficult to identify.

These food allergy also worsen the symptoms of eczema, asthma and rhinitis.

Fortunately, there are actually many subtle telltale signs that most people, even doctors, are not aware of.

If your child with ADHD also has asthma, eczema (atopic dermatitis), and frequent ear infections, there's a very likely chance that he or she has cow's milk sensitivity.

Telltale signs of hidden food allergy in kids with ADHD:

- picky eater (not because of ADHD medication)
- constipation
- diarrhea
- stomach ache
- cramps
- bloating
- nausea
- vomiting
- acting silly or hyper after eating certain food
- craves or addicted to certain types of food
- aggression and agitation
- asthma
- eczema
- ear infection
- dark circles around eyes
- nasal congestion
- coughing or wheezing

If you or your child shows any of the above symptoms with no clear explanation, chances are hidden food allergy may be the reason behind.

If your child has any of these symptoms, an elimination diet should definitely be part of the natural ADHD treatment.

I know. No one wants to change their diet, especially if your child is already picky with food. And who wants to stop eating their favorite foods?

But this step is the most crucial because the elimination diet is not just a trial test diet, it is a therapeutic diet. Eliminating all the potentially harmful trigger food gives the body a break to heal itself.

This means that after the body healed with the elimination diet, your child may be able to tolerate more food than before.

Just taking vitamin supplements without making the necessary diet and lifestyle changes is like taking poison and antidote together everyday.

It's just a matter of time that the body breaks down and not able to recover.

The good news is about 10% of children with ADHD may be able to completely resolve all ADHD symptoms by simply eliminating the problem food additives and food allergens.

For 20-30% of children may achieve partial symptoms resolution. But that does not mean the elimination diet does not work.

It just means there are a few more things to fix, such as nutrition deficiency or digestion issues.

Here's the fun part.

What Foods Do You Eliminate for ADHD?

The *Eat to Focus Diet Protocol* is based on a clean eating concept that focuses on whole natural foods while eliminating most processed, manufactured foods, and fast foods.

Do you know what you are eating and feeding your child every day?

The cruel truth is artificial food additives are everywhere in our food and can affect your child with ADHD tremendously. These artificial food additives provide no health benefit and are used by food manufacturers purely to entice children to eat more processed food AND to make the food last longer than its natural life span to avoid cost from spoilage.

As consumers, of course, we like our food to look delicious. Food manufacturers know very well that we eat with our eyes first. And of course, who doesn't like tasty, delicious meals.

Manmade food additives interacts with our body and brain functions.

Imagine a hostage situation...and you wonder why your child is not acting like himself or herself.

They're not in control, something else is in control.

Think of your body like your own home. How often do you take out your trash?

If you keep bringing garbage into your house and not clean or take out the trash, what would your home look like?

Speaking of which, why would you even bring garbage into your home the first place?

Treat your body like how you would with your home.

Most processed mass-produced food are loaded with toxic ingredients, such as artificial food additives, artificial food coloring, artificial sugars and sweeteners (high fructose corn syrup, Splenda, Equal, Sweet n Low), monosodium glutamate MSG, trans fat and preservatives that damage brain cells and brain chemistry.

Not to mention, ***almost all processed foods are stripped off of essential nutrients for the body and brain***. So basically these are empty calories, that's why people are gaining weight on processed food.

If it comes in a box or package and has a shelf life longer than your pet goldfish, you should not eat it. These are the foods that cause sensitivities in the highest percentage of people.

Many food colorings and high fructose corn syrup that are used in the United States today are banned in many European countries years ago due to documented hyperactivity in children after consumption. We are way behind in the United States.

It also focus on eliminating potential food allergies. The most common food allergies seen in kids with ADHD are cow's milk and gluten. We also eliminated the most common food allergies in the general population - eggs, soy, peanut, and tree nuts. And we'll also eliminated the common harmful GMO crops - grains, corn and beans.

The elimination diet for ADHD should consists of as few food as possible to facilitate symptom relief and identify trigger foods.

1. The "C" Food Snacks

I call these "C" food - cereal, cookies, chips, crackers, cake, chocolate candies, and candies are food that many children eat every day.

The choice for these foods is all driven by food manufacturers and their witty advertising that entice children to choose them over healthy natural choices.

These packaged processed food are loaded with highly processed flours, high fructose corn syrup, trans fat, artificial food colorings, monosodium glutamate, preservatives, other toxic additives, and many more that you don't want to know.

And how these affect your child's brain?

Other than a quick burst of energy from the sugar and carb content, then a sugar crash. If your child tends to have "hangry" issues and emotional meltdowns, take a look at what they're snacking on.

The body needs calming neurotransmitters, such as serotonin and GABA, to calm down. Eating sugar and processed food all day does not give your body any resources to make these neurotransmitters.

2. Bottled Juices, Flavored Drinks, and Diet Drinks

Bottled juices and flavored drinks are just the same as the last category.

Many sodas, flavored drinks, and even sports drinks are flavored with artificial flavorings and high fructose corn syrup and get their pretty color from artificial food coloring.

Diet drinks are no better at all. Diet or sugar-free foods and drinks are not healthier either.

Diet soda and flavored water are advertised as "healthy" alternatives to sugary drinks and pops. But in reality, they are poisonous.

Diet soda and artificially flavored water are contaminated with food colorings, artificial flavorings, and artificial sweeteners to make it tastes sweet and look pretty to drink.

In addition to all the above, diet beverages are sweetened with artificial sweeteners. They are filled with artificial sweeteners, which is poisonous to the body.

But the look is deceiving because these drinks also have no nutritional values other than the toxic burden it adds to your body.

The initial studies that showed artificial sweeteners are safe are sponsored by manufacturers who produce artificial sweeteners. Besides, these studies were done on grown adults who have a different metabolism than children.

Children are still growing, therefore, the effects of artificial sweeteners on growing bone, muscles, and brain tissues are unknown.

Newer studies show that artificial sweeteners increase the risk of insulin resistance and type 2 diabetes, just like real sugar does. So don't be fooled.

What about 100% juice?

They're just as bad. These juice are manufactured months before getting to supermarket shelves. They're pasteurized, meaning all the beneficial enzymes are dead.

I call these "dead juice." They offer no benefits other than empty calories.

Consuming excessive amounts of fructose may influence dopamine regulation, which affects behaviors in children with ADHD, increase the risk of fatty liver and insulin resistance.

The *American Academy of Pediatrics* recommends limiting all sugar to less than 10% of total calories per day (roughly six teaspoons per day for children ages 2 to 19 years) to support good mental and physical health. In my opinion, that's still too much.

Again, if it comes in a bottle and has a shelf life longer than your pet goldfish, you should not drink it.

3. Fast Food

The highly processed food, such as those found in fast-food restaurants and convenience packaged food, is associated with increased obesity. Remember, people with ADHD are more likely to overeat and become obese.

Highly processed food requires minimal effort for digestion, which means empty calories, such as carbohydrates and sugar, get into the bloodstream in a short burst of times, causing blood sugar and insulin spikes, which results in mood swings and fatigue.

High blood sugar and high insulin levels are also associated with increased fat storage and obesity, which is a risk factor of many cancers.

Trans fats are used in many fast foods and processed food, which increases the risk of cardiovascular disease. High-temperature cooking in fried food increases the production of cancer-causing substances in fast food.

Fat-free food is loaded with processed carbohydrates to replace the fats removing, making these foods just a bad as eating pure sugar.

Margarine or butter-replacement spreads are often one molecule away from being plastic. If you leave them out overnight, bugs won't even eat them. Take the hint.

They are not a healthy choice like manufacturers want you to believe. Margarine and butter-replacement spreads are not food and should not be consumed by any human.

4. Instant Packaged Noodles

Instant noodle is an affordable and convenient meal choice for many. Some people eat them because they're cheap. Kids and college kids like them because they're easy.

I always say nothing comes free or cheap, and convenience comes with a price.

The *monosodium glutamate (MSG)* in instant noodles is reason enough to avoid them.

MSG is an excitotoxin, which means it overexcites your nerve cells to the point of damage or death, causing brain dysfunction and damage to varying degrees — and potentially even triggering or worsening learning disabilities, ADHD, Alzheimer's disease, Parkinson's disease, Lou Gehrig's disease, and more.

Part of the problem is that the free glutamic acid (MSG is approximately 78 percent free glutamic acid) is the same brain chemical that your brain, nervous system, eyes, pancreas, and other organs use to initiate specific processes in your body.

Yes, MSG is also the ingredient that makes you want to eat more, and pack on the weight, causing obesity.

5. Canned Goods

Have you ever wonder how canned goods can stay on the shelf for many years, and the metal can never rust?

The magic (or poison) is bisphenol A (BPA). It's the plastic lining that protects the metal can from exposure to the food item to prevent rusting. Bisphenols are also used to harden plastic containers.

BPA is also an endocrine or hormone disruptor and can act like estrogen in the body and potentially change the timing of puberty, affects fertility, increase body fat, and affect the nervous and immune systems. It interferes with the body's natural hormones and affects brain growth and development even before the baby is born.

The good news is BPA is now banned in baby bottles and sippy cups.

6. Processed, Canned and Cured meat

Processed meats are often cured by adding sodium nitrite, which gives them a pink color and a distinct taste, or by adding sodium nitrite and lactic acid, which provides a tangy taste.

Nitrates/nitrites are used to preserve food and enhance color, especially in cured and processed meats, and stop the growth of dangerous botulism.

But scientists suspect they may be involved in the formation of cancer-causing compounds in the body. These chemicals can interfere with thyroid hormone production and the blood's ability to deliver oxygen in the body. Nitrates and nitrites also have been linked with gastrointestinal and nervous system cancers.

Even small amounts of processed meat intake are associated with an increased risk of colorectal cancer. One slice of bacon a day is all it takes to increase your cancer risk by 18%.

8. Fish and Other Seafood with High Mercury Content

Fish and seafood are excellent sources of protein, omega-3 fatty acids, and zinc. However, not all fish and shellfish are equally safe to eat.

Fish, such as **shark, king mackerel, swordfish, marlin, orange roughy, tilefish and most tuna** are loaded with mercury. Mercury attaches to tissue cells and accumulates over time.

Big predator fish tend to have a higher mercury content because they prey on smaller fish and, as a result, inherit their mercury content.

The same process happens when children consume fish contaminated with mercury.

Your child assumes the mercury content from these fish and seafood, and again, the mercury accumulates in your child's body affecting his or her brain growth, development, and behaviors.

Mercury poisoning affects the brain and nerve tissues, the gut and kidneys.

Do you know who else is at risk?

Unborn fetuses…So pregnant women need to avoid these fish and seafood as much as possible.

9. Cow's Milk and Products Made from Cow's Milk

Cow's milk is for baby cows or calves. Human milk is for human babies. Most animals stop drinking milk as they mature, so why are human children drinking milk from another mammal as they mature?

We are not supposed to drink milk from other animals. We are the only mammal who does it. This often translates to intolerance or an allergic reaction to cow's milk proteins.

Between 2% and 3% of children younger than 3 years old are allergic to cow's milk. We used to think that most children would outgrow their cow's milk allergy by the time they turned 3. But recent study showed that fewer than 20% of children outgrow their cow's milk allergy by age 4. And about 80% of children are likely to outgrow their milk allergy before they are 16.

Studies also showed that cow's milk is loaded with many hormones to include *estrogen, insulin growth factor, prolactin, glucocorticosteroid*.

Up to 60-70% of animal estrogens in the human diet comes from cow's milk and dairy products. Cow's milk contains growth hormones for baby cows (calves) to grow. When humans take in these cow's hormones, bad things can happen because they can disrupt our hormonal signaling.

Most people do not tolerate lactose in milk well. Even if it's seemingly unnoticeable, removing lactose from the diet can make a big difference.

In fact, our pancreas produces lactase, the lactose digestive enzyme, up until the age of two to cover the period where we are really supposed to drink breast milk.

Does your child crave dairy products, such as milk, cheese, and yogurt?

Poorly digested milk protein, casomorphine, interacts with the brain reward center like cocaine and heroin. This milk protein binds to the same brain receptor that morphine binds to, creating addictive behaviors towards dairy products, raging behaviors, irritability, anger, and mood swings.

10. Eggs

Egg is one of the eight most common food allergens affecting approximately 2-3% of the population. It's estimated that as many as 2 percent of children are allergic to eggs. Fortunately, about 70 percent of children with an egg allergy will outgrow their egg allergy by age 16.

Young children who are allergic to uncooked egg but can tolerate baked egg may be more likely to outgrow their egg allergy at an earlier age than young children who react to baked egg.

If you are allergic to chicken eggs, you should also avoid eggs from birds such as ducks, geese, turkeys and quails.

The whites of an egg is the most common cause allergic reactions to egg. If you have an egg allergy, you must avoid all egg components completely (both the egg white and the egg yolk). Even if you aren't allergic to egg yolk proteins, it is impossible to separate the egg white completely from the yolk.

Another reason to avoid eggs is the egg white enzyme, lysozyme. Lysozyme in egg whites can pass through the weak leaky intestinal wall. In normal, healthy individuals, lysozyme is not likely to cause damage to the healthy lining of the gut or cause a substantial immune response.

Lysozyme itself is not an issue. But, it does bind with other proteins, especially egg white protein. Lysozyme from egg white typically passes through the leaky gut wall in large complexes with egg white proteins, triggering the body's immune reaction to eggs white.

11. Grains and Legumes

Does your child with ADHD crave bread, crackers, pasta, etc.?

Although humans have been eating grains for thousands of years, the *wheat we eat today is entirely different from the wheat our ancestors ate, even just one generation back.*

Today's grains are making people sick. More and more scientists are catching on about the connection between today's highly modified grains and chronic digestive and inflammatory illnesses.

Grains, such as wheat, barley, and rye, contain gluten, a tough protein for the human body to digest. This can cause inflammation in the intestine and damage the gut lining leading to malabsorption of nutrients.

The gluten in today's grains causes inflammation, and it is also more addicting, which makes you crave and eat more of it. Even a small amount of gluten can cause leaky gut.

Poorly digested gluten, called gliadorphine, can interact with the brain dopamine system triggering unpleasant behaviors, such as anger outbursts and mood swings.

Gliadorphine acts similarly to morphine and binds to the same receptors in the body, triggering addiction behaviors.

There are also studies showing the association between ADHD and Celiac disease.

Celiac disease is an autoimmune disorder where the immune reaction to eating gluten creates inflammation that damages the small intestine's lining.

In one study, researchers tested 67 people with ADHD for celiac disease. Study participants ranged in age from 7 to 42. A *total of 15% tested positive for celiac disease*, which is far higher than the celiac incidence in the general population, which is about 1%.

Grains and legumes also contain anti-nutrients such as saponins and lectins. These tiny molecules are extremely challenging to intestinal defense mechanisms. They open the tight junctions in your gut and make you very sick if you consume them raw.

Eating lectins can damage the intestines and cause leaky gut. As a result, it sets off an allergic reaction that damages the intestinal wall even more and causes more inflammation.

They can also be transported through the damaged intestinal wall into the bloodstream, where they may bind to insulin receptors and leptin receptors.

Lectins also cause leptin resistance, which means that your hunger signal is suppressed and that you'll be hungry even when your body has had more than enough calories.

Grains and legumes also contain phytic acid (phytates) that interfere with food digestion and absorption. Because phytate is formed when phytic acid binds to minerals—typically calcium, magnesium, iron, potassium, and zinc—these minerals are then unavailable to be absorbed by the gut. Therefore, the consumption of phytate-rich foods like grains and legumes can cause mineral deficiencies, especially when these phytate-rich foods displace other mineral-rich foods in the diet.

Phytic acid literally binds to essential minerals, such as magnesium, zinc, iron, and calcium, which are already low in kids with ADHD.

Grains and legumes are poor sources of bioavailable nutrients compared to meat, seafood, vegetables, and fruits. There is not much in grains and legumes that you can't get more potently and healthily from animals or vegetables.

Beans and legumes don't have much to make up for. They can't match the micronutrient content of animal foods, so there isn't any compelling reason to eat them.

Plant sterol in soy attaches to the same estrogen receptors in the body and causes the same effect as it is your body's own estrogen. Therefore, ***males should avoid soy milk,*** and ***women with a family history of breast cancer should avoid soy milk*** too. People with milk allergy should avoid soy as well.

Soy is in a lot of products, too, so when you remove all processed packaged food, you'll eliminate a lot of unnecessary and harmful ingredients in your diet.

Corn (also a grain) is a challenging crop to grow without jacking it up with chemicals. So when you eat corn, you are actually eating those chemicals.

Also, corn has been bred so many times over the years to resist pests. This practice, unfortunately, bred into corn, a compound called fucosamine, which can cause cancer.

The protein in corn is very similar to that in wheat and wheat-like grains. So corn is as damaging to the intestine as grains and can also induce immune and inflammation response.

It is almost impossible to find a clean source of corn these days as 80% of corn and soy grown in the United States are GMO.

My advice....just don't eat corn and soy.

Eating grains, beans, and legumes regularly may be more harmful than healthful.

12. Nuts

Tree nut allergy is one of the eight most common food allergies, affecting roughly 0.5 to 1% of the U.S. population. A true tree-nut allergy means the body produces IgE antibodies against proteins in nuts.

However, preliminary scientific studies show that tree nut intolerance, where the body produces IgG antibodies against proteins in nuts, may affect up to 20 to 50% of the population.

Tree nuts include almonds, Brazil nuts, cashews, hazelnuts, pecans, pistachios, and walnuts.

People who are allergic to tree nuts are often allergic to more than one type of tree nut because many tree nuts are closely related, such as cashew with pistachio, and pecan with walnut.

Also, being allergic to one tree nut does not necessarily mean you are allergic to other tree nuts. It may be appropriate and safe to eat certain tree nuts while avoiding others.

Thirty percent of individuals who are allergic to peanuts are also allergic to tree nuts. However, having a tree nut allergy does not necessarily mean you are allergic to peanuts too.

People who are allergic to tree nuts can usually tolerate seeds such as sesame, sunflower seeds, and pumpkin seeds without difficulty.

The term "nut" does not always indicate a tree nut. Nutmeg, water chestnut, butternut squash, and shea nuts are not tree nuts. Macadamia nuts and pine nuts are actually seeds. Therefore, they're generally well tolerated by people with a tree nut allergy.

People with a tree nut allergy can also tolerate coconut without difficulty because coconut is not truly a nut but rather a fruit. Tigernuts are not nuts. they are small tubers, like sweet potato, though much smaller in size.

Tree nut allergy typically starts in childhood and persists throughout life; approximately 10% of individuals may outgrow tree nut allergy over time.

13. Dirty Dozen

Each year the *Environmental Working Group (EWG)* publishes a fresh list of produce highly contaminated with pesticides.

Pesticides were originally invented as a nerve gas to use as biological weapons during war. Since we didn't really have a war to use this technology, why waste it. Let's use it to kill pests.

Who knows these pesticides are leaking into the food system and affecting our children and adults?

Organophosphates create the same action as nerve gases such as sarin and are one of the most widely used classes of pesticides in the U.S. and around the world.

They inhibit the cholinesterase, an enzyme in the human nervous system that breaks down the neurotransmitter acetylcholine, which carries signals between nerves and muscles.

When cholinesterase is inactivated, acetylcholine builds up in the nerves. Victims die from suffocation because their lungs are paralyzed, and they can't breathe.

A study published in the journal *Pediatrics* showed that legally permissible amounts of organophosphates have extraordinary effects on brain chemistry.

The findings concluded that *children with above-average pesticide exposures are two times more likely to have ADHD, indicating the build-up of acetylcholine in the nerves that causes over-activity.*

14. Genetically Modified Organism Food

Genetically modified food is not entirely unknown to humans. Humans have domesticated plants and animals since around 12,000 BCE using selective breeding or artificial selection, which is the opposite of Darwinian's natural selection.

In selective breeding, the organisms with desired traits or genes are used for breeding the next generation, and organisms with the undesired trait or genes are not reproduced. This is a precursor to the modern genetic modification.

Real-life example – dog breeding. Therefore, farmers and agricultural scientists have been genetically engineering the foods we eat for centuries through selective breeding programs.

The new generation of genetically modified organisms (GMOs), on the other hand, are living organisms whose genetic material or DNA has been artificially manipulated in a laboratory through genetic engineering. This creates combinations of plant, animal, bacteria, and virus genes that do not occur in nature or through traditional crossbreeding methods.

Food is modified to a form that our body cannot recognize. Therefore, it stimulates our immune system to overreact. GMOs have also been shown to cause cancer through cellular damages.

Other ways to minimize exposure to environmental toxins:

- Use glass or stainless steel containers instead of plastic containers for food or beverage to avoid BPA exposure.
- Do not heat food in plastic containers in the microwave. The high temperature causes the BPA to be released into the food.
- Avoid bottled water and plastic water bottle. Install a whole house water filter system if you can afford one.
- Cook food in aluminum cookware. Avoid non-stick Teflon surface
- Avoid reusable plastic bottles or containers labeled 3 and 7
- Avoid Genetically Modified Organism (GMOs)
- Avoid these 9 Artificial Food Coloring: Erythrosine (red #3), Allura Red AC (E129) (FD&C Red #40, Red 40), Ponceau S (E124, Acid Red 112), Carmoisine (E122, Acid Red 14), Sunset yellow (E110) (FD&C; Yellow #6), Tartrazine (E102) (FD&C; Yellow #5), Quinoline yellow (E104) – Yellow coloring, Brilliant Blue (FD & C Blue #1), Fast Green (FD&C Green #3, Green 1724)#2 (E133)

Stay on this *Clean Start Phase* for at least eight weeks to give the body enough time to clear out all toxins and inflammation and recover.

Use the **Food Intake and Symptom Trackers** in the *Appendix* to help you track progress and identify potential trouble food.

PHASE 2

FEED THE ADHD BRAIN

"Real food doesn't have ingredients. Real food is ingredients." - Jamie Oliver

I apologize for all the bad news in the last section. But I hope to help you see that many of the so-called "healthy foods" are not that safe for our body and that some of your child's ADHD symptoms may be the result of eating those foods for years.

Now that we got all the junk and poison out the system, are you wondering what food to feed your child today?

I'm so excited about this diet because it's the best ADHD diet in the world. You get to eat all the delicious and HEALTHY foods on this diet.

When we give the body what it needs with the right kind of human food, we can then *see how the body functions in its true self*, and see the real signs and symptoms without the influence of toxic food additives and inflammation.

When you nourish your body with the right food and nutrition the way God made them, you'll nourish your body, mind, and soul. You'll feel better mentally and physically.

I always ask my patients about their energy levels. They usually tell me something like "it's good" or "it's normal" or "I feel fine. "

And when they come back at the next visit after making changes to their diet, they respond with "I have so much more energy," "I can run faster," "I think more clearly in my head," "I'm not as tired" or "I want to work out again after working out."

What happened here?

It's called "*the body finally got what it needs*".

Can I Just Take a Multivitamin?

Short cut means short term…How long do you want the results to last?

Many people tried to skip the diet change step and go straight to supplements …that'll work too.

BUT…big but.

If you don't correct any underlying toxic food ingestion, food intolerances or allergies, nutrient deficiencies, you'll be forever dependent on whatever supplements to keep your body functioning.

It's like eating poison every day while also take the antidote. It's just not going to work for long.

Over time, you'll need a higher dose of the supplement to do the same job because you are trying to overcome a function that's handicap or defective that is getting worse over time because of non-treatment.

Supplements are excellent when used as "crutches" while your child's body heals naturally with simple, pure food.

Step 2 aims to feed the body what it needs and correct any nutrient deficiencies while supporting natural healing and normal growth in young children.

What Food Feeds the ADHD Brain?

Have you ever wonder how your baby comes all the way from only eating, pooping and sleeping to walking, crawling, climbing, talking, throwing, and pulling the dog's tail in just 12 short months?

During the first year, the brain develops super fast. You see, your child goes from a baby into a toddler in just under one year.

This is why we always say the baby's brain is like a sponge. It absorbs new knowledge and develops new skills very quickly.

Amazing...

So parents often ask, "What's the best vitamins for the brain?"

The answer is FATS...DIETARY FATS.

The infant brain doubles in weight by two years of age from birth and continues to develop rapidly until at least five years. And the brain does not stop development and reshaping until we die.

As the brain develops more nerve cells, more fat is needed in the form of fatty acids. Each brain cell has a fatty coat outside to protect the brain cell from misfiring. This is called the myelin sheath. It's very much like the plastic casing of electrical wiring. A lot of this is happening in babies and little kids.

Because of these special needs in infants and young children, babies and children need to eat a lot of fat. Up to 50% of calories in their diet should be coming from fats.

We're talking about healthy fats, such as avocado, olive oil, organic animal fats, organic egg yolks, coconut oil, and organic nut are encouraged.

The little *3 pounds human brain accounts for only about 2% of the average adult body weight but eats up to 20% of the daily energy.*

Even though the brain is 60% fat, it functions more like a muscle. It *uses a humongous amount of energy when being used productively.* You know the headache you have after long hours of "brain workout" aka studying or sustained focus.

Are you ready to load up on brain-boosting food for your family' and enjoy a calmer peaceful, no drama life?

Our brain prefers glucose or sugar as the primary source of energy, but in a very rare unusual situation, it *can switch to use fat for energy*.

And children with ADHD have a defect that makes it difficult to use sugar efficiently for brain function. Many children with ADHD *struggle with mood swings and anger issues because of this defect*. The underlying cause can be as simple as the brain not getting the fuel it needs for energy.

The goal of an ADHD diet is to feed the brain the right resources it needs to function properly, balance blood sugar, and correct nutrient deficiency and free of brain-alternating toxins.

Children with ADHD tend to have more poor diets. Studies have shown *children with ADHD consume more refined grains and less calcium and vitamin B's* compared to their non-ADHD counterparts.

As a result, children with ADHD also have more nutrient deficiencies, such as iron, magnesium, zinc, omega-3 fatty acids, vitamin B's, and vitamin D.

Studies also showed that these nutrient deficiencies affect brain functions and behaviors. Therefore, proper food and nutrition intake is essential in controlling ADHD symptoms. And *nutrient supplements may be needed to correct deficiencies and help improve brain functions and ADHD behaviors.*

Studies consistently show ADHD children who suffer from more significant nutrient imbalances have more severe symptoms. Fortunately, with appropriate integrative treatments that restore nutrient deficiencies, children can achieve relief from behavioral symptoms, including inattention, hyperactivity, impulsivity, and oppositional behavior.

Here are the **3 Simple Steps to Replenish the Brain Power**:

1. Eat Simple Pure Food

When I say real food, I mean food that grew out of the ground or fell off of a tree that grew out of the ground or came from an animal that peed on the tree while it was standing on the ground. That food doesn't include ingredients that were created in a laboratory.

It's just simple pure food.

Do you really think your body recognizes squirt cheese from a can as real food?

I know a package out of the vending machine is convenient and it's cheap. But you're going to pay for it one way or the other. You can either spend your money on real food now, or you can pay later in the form of time and effort dealing with an angry child, or taking time off from work to pick up your child early from school because he or she is having a "bad day".

Every meal you eat that is made of real food is giving your body nutrients it can actually use to function and thrive.

Every meal you eat that is made from processed, chemical-ridden ingredients that you can't pronounce, is giving your body a problem it has to deal with.

In the *Eat to Focus Protocol*, you'll be eating the way people ate for most of human history — there's plenty of food that doesn't come from a factory or an industrialized farm. Of course, if you have an intolerance to any of these foods, don't eat it just because it's on this list.

Eating real food means eating nothing processed in any way. It doesn't mean you cannot eat any processed food ever. It's just that the body has a harder time dealing with these junk processed food when it has been overwhelmed for a long time.

When the body is healed and not overwhelmed, eating processed food in small quantity and infrequently will not be as bad.

The *Eat to Focus* diet is nutrient-rich, antioxidant-rich, and toxin-free to promote optimal brain growth and development, enhance the body's detoxification and immune system to reduce inflammation. And also hypoallergenic to avoid unintentional insult to the body.

Choose wholesome natural food made the way God intended for human consumption. Organic non-GMO options are emphasized to ensure that the natural ingredients are without toxic pesticides and genetically altered species.

In the *Eat to Focus* diet plan, nutrition comes mostly from organic animal-based and plant-based foods, such as chicken, beef, lambs, bison, venison, fruits, and vegetables.

Unprocessed whole foods from various plant sources are naturally rich in antioxidants, vitamins, and minerals that provide the nutrients our body needs to function optimally, supporting detoxification processes, reducing inflammation, and boost immunity.

The diet should also provide an adequate amount of dietary fat to feed the brain and provide essential building material for new healthy brain tissues.

Because young children's brains are still growing, introducing healthy fats and a whole food plant-based diet will hopefully improve many of the ADHD symptoms as new healthy brain tissues and connections form.

Besides, healthy fats are packed with essential fat-soluble vitamins, such as vitamin A, vitamin D, vitamin E, and vitamin K, that are super important for normal body function and growth.

Eat real food, such as organic animal protein, organ meats, low glycemic index fruits, and vegetables.

Choose organic animal products (beef, pork, lamb, bison, venison, poultry, seafood, eggs) and organic produce to minimize exposure to toxic antibiotics, pesticides, and growth hormones.

Foods to Eat More Often

1. Organic meats

Animal protein is a good source of cholesterol, which helps to stabilize serotonin receptors. Too low cholesterol levels, serotonin cannot do its job, and ADHD symptoms show up.

Whenever possible, choose meat from grass-fed, free-roaming, and hormone-free animals. You don't even need to eat lean cuts. Animal fats can be very beneficial when your digestion is working properly.

Eat the whole egg, including the yolk, in moderation if you tolerated it after the elimination period. You can even have more than two a day, from free-range chickens. You can eat eggs every day.

There is NO scientific evidence to show the current recommendation of 300mg cholesterol comes from. It was made up by the sugar industry 40-50 years ago to get people to stop eating meat and eggs for breakfast, so people would start eating sugary cereal for breakfast instead.

Choose hormone-free and antibiotic-free beef (grass-fed), chicken, bison, pork, lamb, turkey, and wild game if possible. Chicken has high omega-6 content, so eat in moderation, and if you eat more chicken, then make sure to eat a lot of omega-3 oils to compensate.

Best choices are locally-raised grass-fed and pastured meats. Second, the best is organic. Avoid factory-farmed meats that contain antibiotics and hormones.

If conventionally raised meats (meat from animals that are not grass-fed, hormone-free, free-roaming animals) is your only option, then you should always eat the lean cuts and avoid fats.

Animals store their toxins in fat tissues, so if an animal is pumped full of antibiotics and other harmful chemicals, you don't want to eat that animal's fat where much of those toxins are stored.

2. Organ meats

Organ meats, such as connective tissue, organs, joints, skin, and bone broth, are excellent sources of elastin, collagen, and glycine, which are great for healing leaky gut.

Elastin and collagen are the most abundant protein in the human body. Collagen makes up most of the connective tissue in your body. It's essential for ***keeping muscles, bones, and connective tissues strong and stable.***

Glycine is an amino acid that makes up about 1/3 of the elastin and collagen, making one of the most abundant amino acids in the body.

Glycine helps maintain healthy levels of acidity in the digestive tract and also breaking down fatty acids.

As a brain chemical, *glycine is calming and helps improve memory and learning.* Studies showed supplementing the diet with glycine helps improve memory and attention span in young adults. Glycine supplement also seems to fall asleep easier.

Try to have organ meats or collagen bone broth at least x5 times a week. Drink a cup of homemade bone broth every morning or use a collagen powder in your morning smoothie or breakfast bowl.

3. Wild Caught Seafood

Fish and seafood are excellent sources of zinc, selenium, vitamin D, and omega-3 fatty acid, all of which are major brain nutrients.

As the brain develops more nerve cells, and more fat, in the form of fatty acids, is needed. And o**mega-3 fatty acid makes up about 8-10 percent of brain tissues**. It is the major component of myelin sheaths on nerve cells.

Wild-caught cold-water fatty fish, such as *salmon, mackerel, haddock, trout, flounder, sardines*, blue crab, and shrimps are your best bet. *Wild-caught seafood is least contaminated by industrial mercury, pesticides, antibiotics, and growth hormone.*

Encourage your pregnant friends to take omega-3 fatty acid supplements. *Studies showed pregnant women who take omega-3 fatty acids during pregnancy, their children have a lot lower risk of developing ADHD.*

4. Low Glycemic Index Fruits and vegetables

Most people eat a diet loaded with carbohydrates (both good and bad), which eventually turn to sugar that feeds not just our brain but also some unwelcome guests in our intestine – yeast or candida unfriendly bacteria.

Eat slow-carb or low glycemic index food and *avoids all simple and processed carbohydrates may help to balance blood sugar levels. It may also help to prevent and treat candida and bacterial overgrowth.*

Choosing more slow carbs and fruits and vegetables prevents blood sugar spikes, stimulating the dopamine reward center in the brain, and creating sugar addiction and cravings.

The vitamins and minerals in plants help to drive all the biochemical reactions in our bodies. When people *change to a plant-based diet, they feel more energetic, and their brain fog clears up*.

And the *fiber from fruits and vegetables helps to improve bowel health and promote healthy bacteria and prevent leaky gut*.

Dark green vegetables are excellent sources of *vitamin K, calcium, magnesium, and iron*. The green color of vegetables comes from *chlorophyll*, which is the powerhouse of pant. In humans, *chlorophyll is a powerful antioxidant* great for detoxification.

Choose more vegetables than fruits. *Limit low glycemic index fruits to only three servings a day eaten in 3 separate times throughout the day to avoid sugar highs and the following sugar crash.*

Always eat fruits with a protein or fats, such as apple slices with chicken slices, grapes with chicken cubes, or fresh berries with coconut milk yogurt.

5. Fermented Foods

Before you get all gross-out, hear me out first.

Fermented foods are food that has been exposed to natural, good bacteria called lactobacilli. The bacteria feed on the starches and sugars in the food and convert them to this tangy and sour-tasting lactic acid.

This process is called *fermentation,* which also makes essential vitamin Bs, magnesium, and zinc, more available. And *these are the same nutrients that can improve focus, memory, and mood.*

Besides, making essential nutrients more available, these bacteria in the intestine also makes amino acids, such as *phenylalanine, tyrosine, and tryptophan,* which the intestine uses to communicate with the big brain on the shoulder. You'll learn more about it in the upcoming section.

Try to eat at least one fermented food or beverage every day.

6. Healthy Unprocessed Fats

The ADHD brain does not process carbohydrates or sugar very efficiently. Therefore, a *lower carb (mainly processed carbs and sugar) and a higher fat diet are more suitable.*

The idea is that *supplying the brain with different fuel sources might boost brain function,* such as focus, memory, and processing speed.

Healthy fats include avocado, avocado oil, coconut oil, coconut cream, extra virgin olive oil, nuts, seeds, pasture-raised/grass-fed animal fats, and fatty cold-water fish.

Avoid processed vegetable oils, such as canola oil, vegetables, oil, etc.

7. Coconut

You've probably heard of *coconut oil's benefits in reserving some of the symptoms of Alzheimer's disease*. This is how it works.

Coconut oil is an excellent source medium-chain triglycerides, or MCTs, which are metabolized very differently than other types of fat in the body. The MCTs in coconut oil eventually break down into ketones, which can be used by the brain cells for fuel.

Coconut oil is also a good source of caprylic acid, a potent anti-fungal, which literally "pokes holes" in the yeast cell wall and kills it.

Choose whole coconut products, such as coconut butter, coconut cream, coconut flakes and chips, unsweetened coconut yogurt, fresh coconut, which may have high inulin fiber.

8. Herbs and spices

Herbs and spices are excellent sources of antioxidants that can help the body function more efficiently. Theses include basil, Celtic salts, cilantro, cinnamon, coriander, clove, garlic, ginger, Hawaiian sea salt, horseradish, Himalayan pink salt, lemongrass, mace, mint, oregano, parsley, rosemary, sage, saffron, sea salt, thyme, turmeric, black pepper, etc.

9. Natural Sweeteners

Unlike other sugar alternatives, stevia and monk fruit contain zero calories and does not impact your blood sugar.

Stevia sweeteners come from the leaves of the stevia rebaudiana (Bertoni) plant, an herbal shrub native to South America. The stevia plant has been used for food and medicinal purposes for hundreds of years.

Monk fruit gets its sweetness from the natural antioxidants in the fruit. It has a glycemic index of zero and can be used as a 1:1 substitute for sugar.

I suggest using *only 100% organic stevia and monk fruit in powdered leaf or liquid extract form.* Avoid products mixed with sugar alcohol or natural flavors and other added chemicals.

2. Eat Slow Carbs

The problem is not so much their ADHD brain, but the food they eat throughout the day.

When someone mentions "snacks," what comes to your mind?

Cookies, candies, chips, crackers, cakes, chocolate, soda pops, right?

What do all these snacks have in common?

Right...processed carbs and sugar.

Everything that you eat and drink affects your body in various ways. It is essential to understand that what you eat can have an immediate effect on your energy and blood sugar levels, which affect you mentally and physically.

Normally, when you eat carbs or sugar, your body reacts with producing insulin, which pushes the sugar into cells for energy.

However, when you consume carbs or sugar in large quantities, your body overacts with making too much insulin, forcing the sugar into cells too fast. This results in a sudden drop in blood sugar, which many people are familiar with the "sugar crash."

This "sugar crash" can be blamed for many mood swings and temper tantrums.

Is your child hungry for food all the time? And here's why.

The other issue with this scenario is that the insulin remains high until your next carb-loaded meal or snack, which keeps the insulin high all day. When insulin level is up, it blocks stored fat from being used as energy.

The body is supposed to use stored fat between meals for energy. The same reason why you don't die in your sleep because of not eating. Now your sugar level tanks and you can't use stored fat for energy. Do you see why people can get "hangry"?

So you binge on more carbs...and because the high insulin level is blocking fat from being used, you can't use stored energy, and you keep eating.

I'm not saying you should stop eating sugar and carbs altogether. But learn to choose wisely because not all carb is the same.

There are simple vs. complex carbs, fast carbs vs. slow carbs, and bad vs. good carbs. Keep reading to see which one is best for your child.

Fast Carbs vs. Slow carbs

Fast carbs cause blood sugar spikes, followed by a blood sugar crash, which we call the ***blood sugar roller coaster***, the reason behind "mood swings" after eating sugary food.

This is what you would use to correct low blood sugar. A pure sugar that gets into the bloodstream fast, 15 minutes or less.

Slow carbs enter the bloodstream slowly and evenly, giving the body plenty of time to clear the sugar from the blood and keep blood sugar level even, which keeps your mood even as well. And it promotes fat burning.

After soda and candies, processed fruit juice is the next worst thing for your body.

For children, it fills up your child's belly, so they're not hungry for real food at mealtimes. Then they become overweight because all they do is drink juice all day long.

For adults, it just another source of unnecessary calories.

Parents frequently tell me proudly that they serve their children "organic 100% juice" like it is the thing that only a good parent would do.

But I'm sorry to burst your bubble and let you know that fruit juices (including your organic 100% juice) are the worst drink for anyone.

These processed organic 100% juice is no different than soda. They're both just sugar and water. With the high temperature for pasteurizing, most essential nutrients of live plants, "live enzymes" are all destroyed.

If you want to include juice as part of a healthy diet, this juice needs to be unprocessed made from fresh organic produce consumed within an hour of making and contain mostly vegetables.

Also, the other use of fruit juice is for treating constipation in young children. And all you need is a couple of ounces of undiluted fresh juice.

If your juice is shelf-stable, it's sugar water. Don't be fooled.

Shelf-stable food is great…for the manufacturers. It gives them longer time for transportation to local stores and a longer time on the shelf to sell.

Bottomline…higher profit margins for manufacturers. Zero health benefits of consumers.

If your kids have aggression, anger issues, and mood swings, the first thing to check is their diet and remove as many empty carbs as possible.

I'm not saying your child needs to eat *no carbs*. Your child needs a steady stream of *"slow carbs" from low or moderate carb food*.

Another reason sugar is hurting your child is that the *fluctuation in blood sugar can cause inflammation throughout the body and trigger unnecessary immune responses that further compromised the brain function of the ADHD brain*.

When you removed most of those junk carb, your blood glucose becomes more stable, and so is your mood. Many people who eat a lower carb diet report better energy and better moods.

These peaks and troughs of blood glucose cause some of the anger outbursts and emotional meltdowns seen in kids with ADHD. Their little body is just trying to regular itself.

Think Hangry. They are the same idea.

The goal of snacks between meals is to help stabilize blood sugar until the next meal.

Children are growing rapidly, so they need to eat a little more often than adults, especially young children. But not let them graze all day long. It's not good for the liver or the immune system.

Many families are pleasantly surprised to discover that many food cravings and addictions disappear once they remove most of the food their child is reacting to, stabilize blood sugar, and replace diet with more nutrient-dense real foods.

You'll find the complete list of *foods to avoid* and list of *foods to eat every day* in the APPENDIX at the end of the book.

3. Correct Nutrient Deficiencies

I always believe eating real whole foods is the best way to get all the vitamins, minerals, and antioxidants your body needs. But you cannot correct a nutrient deficiency with food alone. And this is when you need to hire help.

Supplements are a great way to take a high dose of the deficient nutrient in one single pill. Think of it as your "cheat pill."

Instead of eating a bucket of greens to get the magnesium and iron you need, you only need to swallow one tiny pill.

One caveat: These supplements only work if your child follows a clean, healthy whole food plant-based diet.

Your child's brain is powered by vitamins, minerals, and antioxidants, not empty calories. We'll talk about these vitamins and minerals soon.

Supplements are usually meant for short term use until the underlying nutrient deficiency is corrected.

Correcting your child's unique nutritional imbalances is an integral part of treating his or her ADHD symptoms. Minerals and vitamins are needed for both physical and mental health.

Are you still experimenting with natural supplements to see what works for your child's ADHD?

There are many reasons why ADHD supplements you tried did not work. Keep reading, and you'll learn how to treat ADHD naturally based on your child's needs.

In my practice, I usually help parents develop a diet and supplement regimen based on their constitutional symptoms to reduce ADHD symptoms. That way, *they can either avoid starting ADHD medication or need fewer ADHD medications, which, in turn, means fewer side effects.*

Children's brains are continuous growing and developing. Therefore, the purpose of supplementation is to focus on correcting any nutrient deficiency while supplying the body with the proper nutrition so the brain can grow new healthy brain cells and develop better neuronal connections.

The idea is that if we get our kids the right nutrients to build better brain tissue and connection while learning new skills, hopefully, the ADHD symptoms will improve, and your child may even outgrow ADHD by adulthood.

While loading the body with nutrients from a clean eating plan, we're also detoxifying the body simultaneously.

Remember, *most of the supplements I'm recommending in this book are essential vitamins, minerals, and nutrients that our body needs for basic survival and thrive.*

So these are *nothing special or fancy, but the results are magical*. And they don't cost an arm or a leg.

In conventional medicine, we're so used to the "medicine" idea that one pill is for one disease or one symptom.

However, with functional or holistic medicine, you may be able to correct multiple problems with just one supplement.

For instance, magnesium is responsible for over 300 biochemical reactions in the body. So correcting a magnesium deficiency will result in some pretty significant outcomes.

Another time I saw a teenage girl because she suddenly started losing weight for no reason. She had worked up for everything under the sun and saw all the specialists we have in the hospital. Everything came back normal. The only other complaint she has was body aches and extreme fatigue.

She couldn't even sit up straight in the chair. She slumped in the chair, closed her eyes to take a break in the middle of conversations. She just looked miserable for a teenager.

I started her on a double dose ***B-complex (cheap drugstore brand) in the morning***, then again in the afternoon, if she's still tired.

A week later, she returned for follow up with her mom. What a difference? A normal energetic teenager.

Not just that, mom also mentioned that her eczema cleared up as she started the B-complex.

We not only fixed her fatigue, but her eczema cleared up too. That was a pleasant side effect.

Mom told me that many years ago, her daughter was told to take B-complex for something she couldn't remember, and it did clear her eczema back then. They stopped because they're told to stop, and mom just followed what she was told. And eczema returned until now.

So, are you ready for a boost of ADHD supplements to improve focus and memory naturally and other issues too?

Remember the common nutrient deficiencies in kids with ADHD from the previous section. We're going over every single one of them here.

How to Correct Essential Fatty Acid Deficiencies?

As the brain develops more nerve cells, more fat, in the form of fatty acids, is needed. Omega 3 fatty acids make up about 8-10 percent of brain tissues. It is the major component of myelin sheaths on nerve cells. Myelin is the fatty coating on nerve cells.

The myelin sheaths insulate nerve cells (imagine electrical wiring) to ensure the smooth, uninterrupted transmission of impulses, preventing misfiring of nerve impulses. Rapid myelination during early childhood is what helps the brain develops.

Both docosahexaenoic acid (DHA) and eicosapentaenoic acid (EPA), the active forms of omega-3 fatty acids, play essential roles in brain development. **DHA has a structural function**, and **EPA has a functional role** in the brain development.

DHA is the major structural component of nerve cells and also a significant component of the retina in the eye. EPA affects hormone metabolism, dopamine (brain chemical that regulates mood) metabolism, and immune systems.

Fish oil is an excellent source of omega-3 fatty acids, DHA and EPA, while flaxseed oil and algal oil are excellent sources of alpha-linolenic acid (ALA), which is the precursor to DHA and EPA. ALA is an essential fatty acid, which means our body cannot produce this fatty acid. Our body can make DHA and EPA from ALA.

However, our body is not good at converting ALA to DHA and EPA. This is even more so in children with ADHD. Males, in particular, have a harder time converting ALA to DHA and EPA than females.

Not only do children with ADHD have a harder time making DHA and EPA, but studies also show that many children with ADHD have deficient blood levels of omega-3 fatty acids. Therefore, animal-source of DHA and EPA are preferable.

Low levels of essential fatty acids are associated with autism, ADHD, dyslexia, apraxia, depression, and anxiety.

Omega-3 fatty acids are one of the most studied nutrients for ADHD. Its safety record is outstanding. It is even included in most infant formula nowadays and recommended to pregnant and lactating women to help with the baby's visual and brain development.

Researches and studies have shown that omega-3 fatty acids supplementation improves ADHD symptoms, such as hyperactivity, inattentiveness, aggression, anxiety, impulsiveness, and learning difficulties.

Another group of researchers gave omega-3s for 12 weeks to 41 children aged 8-12 years with both specific learning difficulties and above-average ADHD ratings. They found significant improvements on seven out of 14 scales compared with zero for the placebo group.

A 2012 trial using 600mg a day DHA from algal oil found behavioral improvements judged by parents in six of seven scales from a subset of children whose baseline reading skills were in the lowest 20th percentile. The researchers described the DHA as having "modest benefit.

How to Choose the Right Fish Oil Supplements for Your Child with ADHD?

Are you confused with all the choices of fish oil supplements for ADHD available? Fish oil vs. cod liver oil? What's the right dose?

I got all those answers here for you…just keep reading.

I see many parents give their children fish oil for ADHD, but *did not see the results they expected*. What I notice is that many parents are giving the wrong dose, mainly too little.

I called it the "*Sprinkle Dilemma*."

When you give too little of anything, you'll see little or no result because the amount is too small, it's like a drop in the ocean.

With many fish oil or omega-3 fatty acid gummies out there, you may need to take up to 20 gummies a day to get the right dose of omega-3 fatty acid.

I'll show you how to choose the best fish oil supplements with the right dose for your child with ADHD.

How Much Omega 3 Fatty Acid Does a Child with ADHD Need?

There is *no official recommended daily allowance of omega-3 fatty acids.* Most organizations recommend a minimum of 250-500 mg combined EPA (eicosapentaenoic acid) and DHA (docosahexaenoic acid) each day for healthy adults. However, higher amounts are often recommended for specific health conditions.

And children with ADHD need more DHA and EPA than children without ADHD. They may need up to 500mg to 1,000mg DHA from fish oil or cod liver oil.

Most study doses range from *200 to over 500mg EPA*. Studies with *EPA doses of 500mg or more seem to improve hyperactivity symptoms the most.*

What is the difference between Fish Oil, Cod Liver Oil, and Krill Oil?

They are basically the same thing.

Fish oil is the oil extract from fatty fish. Cod liver oil is the oil extract from the liver of cod (cold fatty fish). And krill oil is the oil extract from the tiny krill shrimp.

The benefits of fish oil for ADHD come from omega-3 fatty acids, EPA, and DHA. Most studies focus on whether omega-3 fatty acid benefits ADHD and did not distinguish between the origins of the omega-3.

To me, the choice between cod liver oil, fish oil, and krill oil is more a personal preference like choosing chicken, pork, fish, or beef to get your protein from.

The only difference is that with cod liver oil, you'll get vitamin A and vitamin D because the body stores it's fat-soluble vitamins in the liver. That's why the liver is good brain food along with other organ meats.

In general, I start most of my patients with ADHD on 500mg DHA. And many *report noticeable improvements in attention*.

If your child is experiencing more *emotional problems and anger issues, I will focus more on EPA*.

To find out *how much EPA and DHA is in your child's fish oil supplement*, you first look at the serving size on the top of the nutrition label, and it'll tell you what's the serving size is for the product.

The brands that I recommend the most are [Carlson Cod Liver Oil](#) and [Nordic Naturals ProOmega 2000](#).

In Carlson's, a serving is one teaspoon or 5ml. If you scroll down the nutrition label, you'll find that it has 4.5 grams of Norwegian Cod Liver Oil, 1,100mg omega-3 fatty acids. And within the 1,100mg omega-3 fatty acids are 500mg of DHA and 400mg EPA. Plus, some vitamin A, vitamin D, and vitamin E.

In Nordic Naturals ProOmega 2000, a serving is 2 capsules per day. If you scroll down the nutrition label, you'll find "Total Omega-3s," Under that, you'll find the amount of EPA and DHA.

In this case, *every 2 capsules of Nordic Naturals ProOmega 2000, you'll get 1,125mg EPA and 875mg DHA*, which is a very decent amount to start with a clean ADHD diet.

Most kids take these with no issues. I like to get the fruity flavors and take mine mixed in yogurt or smoothies.

When I tell parents that their kids need to take **15-20 fish oil gummies a day** of their current gummy vitamins to get the same 500mg omega-3 for better brain functions, their eyes pop wide opened.

To get 250mg DHA, with SmartyPants Kids Formula Daily Gummy Vitamins & Omega 3 Fish Oil, your child will need 23 gummies a day. With OLLY Kids Super Brainy Gummy Multivitamin, your child will need seven gummies a day.

The best fish oil gummy I've found is the [Nordic Omega-3 Fishies](). Your child will need only 2.5 gummy "fishies" a day.

Also, be aware of the sugar content of gummy vitamins.

These are the reason why I recommend against fish oil gummy supplements. So don't waste your money on "gummies."

Can you eat fish to get omega-3?

Yes, you can.

Dr. Weil recommends eating fatty fish x2-3 times a week for general health and a diet low in omega-6 fatty acids.

3oz (150g) of salmon contains 3,200mg fish oil, of which 1,900mg EPA and 1,300mg DHA.

Other good fish choices are *mackerel, seabass, oysters, sardines, herring, shrimp, trouts, and black cod.*

As is almost always the case with all nutrients, nutrients are better absorbed in its natural food form, because that's what our body was created to process. *Whole fish also provides nutrients that fish oil supplements can't.*

But keep in mind, *you cannot correct a nutrient deficiency with food alone.*

There are also a few considerations about getting all of your omega-3s from whole fish.

Many fish are contaminated with toxins, such as PCBs and mercury. Eating the amount of whole fish to meet the therapeutic dose of EPA and DHA could also increase your toxins intake.

While it's always best to get your nutrients from whole foods, *eating wild Alaskan salmon (the most uncontaminated variety) daily can get very expensive.*

While **eating fish** is an excellent source of omega-3 fatty acids, not everyone is a seafood fan. If eating fish is not your thing, high potency fish oil supplements are available, and they're great alternatives to eating fish every day.

How to Correct Magnesium Deficiency?

Can you believe up to 95% of children with ADHD are deficient in magnesium?

Magnesium deficiency signs and symptoms include *sensitivity to loud noises, insomnia, anxiety, hyperactivity, inattentiveness, restlessness, panic attacks, salt craving, and both carbohydrate craving and carbohydrate intolerance.*

Magnesium is involved in over 300 different biochemical reactions in the human body.

Can you imagine being deficient in a mineral that's so important?

Among the 300 functions it does, magnesium is needed for the brain signaling systems. It helps makes serotonin, the calming and feel-good brain chemical. A low level of serotonin is associated with depression, mood swings, and irritability.

Magnesium also calms the nerves by interfering with the release of acetylcholine and catecholamines. Both of these brain chemicals can make you feel anxious and nervous.

Another essential function of magnesium is building myelin sheaths that insulate the nerve cells in the brain. The myelin sheaths are like the plastic casing on electrical wires. This protective layer prevents nerve impulses from misfiring, which can result in seizures.

Magnesium also activates the enzyme that converts dietary alpha-linolenic acids (ALA) into docosahexaenoic acid (DHA), a major component of brain cell membranes.

Green vegetables, nuts, and dark chocolate are excellent sources of magnesium. However, food processing and cooking may deplete magnesium content.

Again, you cannot correct a nutrient deficiency with food alone. You need "cheat pills" or supplements to do the heavy-duty job.

In a study where a group of children with ADHD was supplemented with about 200 milligrams (mg) per day of magnesium for six months, there was "a significant decrease of hyperactivity" compared to children in the control group who did not been receive supplemental magnesium.

In another study, children with magnesium deficiency were randomly given 200mg of magnesium supplement a day plus standard ADHD medication or just conventional ADHD medication alone for eight weeks.

Those who take the magnesium with ADHD medications showed a significant improvement in hyperactivity, impulsivity, inattention, opposition, and conceptual level compared to those taking medication alone.

How to Optimize Benefits of Magnesium Supplements for ADHD?

Children with ADHD are believed to have *lower levels of magnesium inside their blood cells. Vitamin B6 boosts the absorption of magnesium into the cells*. Since vitamin B6 helps improve blood cell levels of magnesium, *supplementing magnesium along with B6, will help with ADHD symptoms*.

The typical dose used in studies for children with ADHD is *200 mg of magnesium and 10 to 20 mg of vitamin B6 (Pyridoxal 5'-phosphate (P5P)) daily*.

One capsule twice a day of [Terry Naturally P-5-P/MAG](#) provides 200mg magnesium glycinate and 20mg P5P.

You can find magnesium supplements in various salt preparations. Multivitamins and minerals generally contain *magnesium oxide, which is less bulky and inexpensive to manufacture. However, it is not soluble in water, which means the body poorly absorbs it*. Magnesium hydroxide in the milk of magnesia is another example of insoluble magnesium salt. Avoid both magnesium glutamate and magnesium aspartate as well.

Oral *magnesium citrate* is inexpensive and relatively well absorbed. Other useful forms of magnesium include *magnesium glycinate, magnesium gluconate, magnesium taurate, magnesium malate, and magnesium chloride*.

Magnesium taurinate, glycinate, or elemental magnesium is the preferred form that is less likely to cause diarrhea. Magnesium aspartate, chloride, lactate, citrate and glycinate are more soluble and easily absorbed in the intestines.

Too much magnesium in a less-absorbable form can cause loose stool. This side effect can be prevented by reducing the amount of magnesium given and providing it in a more absorbable form.

If larger total daily doses of magnesium are required, divide the dose into smaller amounts and give it multiple times throughout the day for better absorption.

Is Magnesium Safe for Children with ADHD?

The safety of magnesium has been well established. Magnesium supplementation is safe compared to the dangerous side effects of ADHD drugs.

Severe overdoses of magnesium are rare in otherwise healthy people. Getting too much magnesium from the diet is not even possible.

It'll take a lot of supplement or laxative medication to get 5,000mg of magnesium per day to cause magnesium toxicity.

Occasionally, a high dosage of magnesium from supplements or medications can cause mild symptoms like diarrhea, nausea, and stomach cramps.

These symptoms are usually temporary and will go away once dosages are reduced or divided into smaller amounts of magnesium given throughout the day.

Magnesium and vitamin B6 complement each other. Therefore, they are usually supplemented together.

Vitamin B6

Vitamin B6 and magnesium have a co-dependent synergistic relationship. While both vitamin B6 and magnesium gets absorbed into the cells, magnesium helps convert vitamin B6 into its active form, pyridoxal 5'-phosphate (P5P), so it can cross the blood-brain barrier, where it helps make neurotransmitters.

Vitamin B6 is a water-soluble vitamin that's involved in making chemicals in the brain. It is needed to convert L-DOPA into dopamine (the reward brain chemical). It also needs to convert glutamate (an excitatory brain chemical) to GABA (*gamma-*aminobutyric acid), a calming chemical. GABA is the neurotransmitter that calms the brain and muscles.

Remember, dopamine is a brain chemical that ADHD medications try to boost. It's needed for cognitive function, such as attention, memory, and problem-solving skills. A deficiency of dopamine in the pre-frontal cortex is associated with attention deficit and memory problems.

The natural forms of vitamin B6 needed to be converted by the liver to the active form that the body needs. People with impaired liver function, celiac disease, older adults, and children with autism and ADHD have difficulty converting vitamin B6 into its active forms. Therefore, supplementing B6 in its active form, is more appropriate and makes it readily available for use by the body.

Children 7-12 years old should aim for 25mg P5P daily and 13 years and older aim for 50mg daily.

The _Terry Naturally P-5-P/MAG/ZN_ is excellent for the little ones. One capsule once a day with just the right amount of P5P, magnesium, and zinc.

For older kids and adults, _Kirkman P5P Magnesium Glycinate_ one capsule once daily will do the trick.

How to Correct Zinc Deficiency?

Children with ADHD often have low zinc levels due to too much copper and lead toxicity. Zinc and copper are needed to create new brain chemicals and are part of our antioxidant defense system that protects cells from free radical damage.

Minerals are essential for normal growth and development, but they must be maintained in an appropriate balance. So just the right amount is needed.

Too much zinc or too much copper is not good for the brain.

Zinc deficiency may cause ***poor or loss of appetite, diarrhea, impaired immune function, poor or retardation of growth***, delayed sexual maturation, eye or skin lesions, delayed wound healing, ***taste abnormalities, and mental lethargy***.

Chelated zinc, such as picolinate, bis-glycinate, and gluconate, are easier on the stomach and absorption.

The *Zinc Picolinte by Throne Research* and *Vegan Liquid Zinc Sulfate by MaryRuth's* are my favorite zinc liquid supplements.

The Zinc Picolinate by Throne Research contains a mixture of different chelated zinc for even easier absorption. And MaryRuth's Vegan Liquid Zinc is a good tasting zinc supplement for the little ones who cannot swallow pills.

Children aged 6 to 11 years can take 15 mg elemental zinc once daily with meals. Children aged 12 and older may take 30 mg of elemental zinc once daily with meals.

To get 15mg elemental zinc, take 1 capsule of Zinc picolinate by Throne Research or 4 ml of MaryRuth's Vegan Liquid Zinc. To get 30mg elemental zinc, double the above.

Zinc not only good for rebalancing the electrolytes in the ADHD brain, but it's also helpful with increasing appetite for picky eaters. It improves digestion as zinc is needed to make stomach acid.

I have used [zinc lozenges](#) for my daughter and patients, who are super picky and sensitive with taste and texture. "Super picky eater" as in they can tell you change the brand of chicken nuggets or the oil you use in a recipe. The zinc lozenges provide about 20mg of zinc per tablet. This is a great start.

How to Correct an Iron Deficiency?

Iron deficiency in children is more concerning than in adults because an iron deficiency in young children can lead to permanently lower intelligent quotient (IQ) score, developmental delays, and behavioral issues. Therefore, early detection and supplementation in children is essential and may help prevent some types of ADHD by positively influencing dopamine neuron development in the early developmental stages.

Did you know drinking too much milk can cause iron deficiency?

Cow's milk triggers immune response and inflammation, but the high calcium content of cow's milk can cause iron deficiency.

People have been brain-washed by the dairy industry's marketing to believe cow's milk products are keys to strong bones. Studies showed otherwise.

In older children, parents are advised to limit their children's cow's milk intake to no more than 24 ounces daily. Cow's milk is a good source of calcium. When your child drinks too much milk, the excessive amount of calcium from milk may block the body from absorbing iron, resulting in iron deficiency anemia.

Iron is an essential mineral involved in brain function because it is a critical cofactor in the making of neurotransmitters or brain chemicals, such as serotonin, norepinephrine, and especially dopamine.

Multiple studies have shown that low serum iron and ferritin (storage iron) are associated with ADHD symptoms in children compared to control children without ADHD. And iron supplementation has also been shown to improve symptoms of ADHD.

Having adequate iron also prevents lead poisoning, which is a possible cause of ADHD symptoms.

Studies have estimated that restless leg symptoms (RLS) in people with ADHD are up 44%. In chidden with RLS and low ferritin level (less than 40ng/mL), iron supplementation was found to be effective in improving ADHD symptoms.

Given the high comorbidity, children with ADHD should be screened for restless leg syndrome.

Anyone with newly diagnosed restless leg syndrome or RLS patients with recent worsening of symptoms should have their serum ferritin levels measured.

Serum iron is *iron swimming freely in the bloodstream*, while **ferritin** is a protein that contains iron and is the primary form of iron stored inside cells. The small amount of **ferritin** that is released and circulates in the blood is a good reflection of the total amount of iron stored in the body.

This present study looked at the effects of iron supplementation on ADHD in children. Twenty-three non-anemic ADHD children (aged 5-8 years) with serum ferritin levels <30 ng/mL were randomized to either oral iron (ferrous sulfate 80mg/day) or placebo for 12 weeks.

There was a significant decrease in the ADHD symptoms in children after 12 weeks on iron supplementation, but not in the placebo group.

Iron supplementation (iron sulfate 80 mg/day) appeared to improve ADHD symptoms in children with low serum ferritin levels.

***80mg iron sulfate = 16mg elemental iron

Floradix Liquid Iron Supplement is an excellent iron supplements that taste great, gentle on the stomach, and easy to absorb. To get the same 16mg elemental iron with Floradix, you'll need to take 15ml a day .

Just a friendly reminder, taking a supplement does not replace a healthy brain-boosting diet.

How to Correct Vitamin B6 Deficiency?

Vitamin B6 is a water-soluble vitamin and one of the vitamin B's that make up the complex. It is found in one of three naturally occurring forms – *pyridoxine, pyridoxal, pyridoxamine*, and three respective 5'-phosphate esters. Pyridoxal 5' phosphate (PLP) and pyridoxamine 5' phosphate (PMP) are the active coenzyme forms of B6 that participate in amino acid metabolism.

Doses of vitamin B6 in research studies averaged 18 mg/kg body weight/day (8 mg/pound daily), which is about 320 mg per day for a 40-pound child.

Studies showed children with ADHD have lower levels of magnesium inside their blood cells. Since B6 helps improve blood cell level of magnesium, supplementing magnesium along with B6, will help with ADHD symptoms.

Magnesium and vitamin B6 have a co-dependent relationship. While B6 boosts the absorption of magnesium into the cells, magnesium is needed for the proper functioning of alkaline phosphatase, which helps the absorption of B6 into the body tissues.

The study mentioned above of young children with an average age of 6-7 years old showed improvement in behaviors, such as inattention, aggressiveness, and hyperactivity with treatment with magnesium and B6.

The amounts used were *6 mg/kg/day magnesium and 0.6mg/kg/day vitamin B6 - roughly 100-200 mg of magnesium and around 10-20 mg of vitamin B6.*

*** see Magnesium section for recommendation.

How to Correct Vitamin B12 Deficiency?

The general recommendation of vitamin B12 is between 0.4 to 2.4 mcg (micrograms) daily, depending on age.

Generally, to treat ADHD, you may start with 1,000 mcg and go up to 2,500mcg per day. Toxicity is rare since Vitamin B12 is water-soluble, which means our body can easily get rid of the extra.

And since people with low vitamin B12 are likely to have gastrointestinal symptoms that interfere with vitamin B12 absorption, the best way to quickly increase and maintain vitamin B12 levels is with vitamin B12 injections, chewable tablets, or the recently released nasal sprays and skin patches.

There are several forms of vitamin B12 – cyanocobalamin, methylcobalamin, and adenosylcobalamin are the physiological or active form.

Cyanocobalamin is the synthetic form that does not occur in nature. It is commonly found in supplements due to its stability and cheaper cost of manufacturing. Theoretically, cyanocobalamine is readily converted to the active forms, methylcobalamin, and adenosylcobalamin in the body.

It also contains about 2% of cyanide or 20 micrograms cyanide in a 1 mg cyanocobalamin tab. This amount may seem minute. However, children with ADHD, as you have read so far, have an inefficient detoxification system. Even a minute amount of cyanide may accumulate over time, causing neural damages.

One of the functions of B12 is methyl donation. Supplementation with cyanocobalamin would not serve this purpose.

Sublingual and spray methylcobalamin are supposedly much easier to absorb because these routes bypass the intestines, which can be an issue for people with GI problems.

Methylcobalamin is the active form, which means the body can use it right away without any further conversion. Besides, children with ADHD just seem to have very different metabolic requirements.

The methylcobalamin supplement from premium brand usually is free of additives, preservatives, artificial colorings, artificial sweeteners, etc. So you are definitely paying for quality for your money.

How to Correct Low Vitamin D Level?

Most people meet at least some of their vitamin D needs through exposure to sunlight. Ultraviolet (UV) B radiation with a wavelength of 290–320 nanometers penetrates bare skin and converts 7-dehydrocholesterol to pre-vitamin D3, which in turn becomes vitamin D3.

Cloudy days can reduce UV energy by as much as 50%, and a shade (including that produced by severe pollution) reduces it by up to 60%. UVB radiation does not penetrate glass, so exposure to sunshine indoors through a window does not produce vitamin D. Sunscreens with a sun protection factor (SPF) of 8 or more appear to block vitamin D-producing UV rays as well.

Fatty fish (such as salmon, tuna, and mackerel) and fish liver oils are among the best sources of vitamin D. Small amounts of vitamin D are also found in beef liver, cheese, and egg yolks. Vitamin D in these foods is primarily in the form of vitamin D3 and its metabolite 25(OH)D3.

There are very few vegan sources of vitamin D in nature. Some mushrooms provide vitamin D2 in variable amounts after being exposed to ultraviolet light under controlled conditions.

Food is always the best source of nutrients. However, when you have a deficiency, food alone cannot correct the deficiency efficiently. Vitamin D supplements are your best bet to correct a confirmed vitamin D deficiency.

Multiple studies showed that vitamin D supplements might improve ADHD symptoms in children who are deficient in vitamin D.

Vitamin D supplements not only improve some behavioral problems but may prevent exacerbation in some symptoms of the disorder and reduce impulsivity.

How Much Vitamin D to Supplement for ADHD?

In a double-blind, parallel clinical trial, 70 students with ADHD (6-13 years old) are given either 1,000IU vitamin D3 supplements or placebo daily for three months.

Another review study of 4 randomized control trials involving 256 children with ADHD. These children are being treated with methylphenidate and vitamin D for a duration of 6 to 12 weeks. The vitamin D doses used were between 1,000 IU per day, and 50,000 IU once a week.

How to Treat MTHFR Defect?

First of all, avoid extra folic acid, the synthetic form of folate. People who have MTHFR gene defect cannot properly use folic acid and often don't feel well after taking it.

Many *B vitamin supplements, multivitamins, energy drinks, protein bars, and processed foods contain synthetic folic acid, and therefore, should be avoided.*

Other forms of folate are generally better for those with MTHFR, including 5-MTHF, methylfolate, and folinic acid.

Of course, you can always get the natural **folate from naturally** folate-rich foods, including spinach, asparagus, chickpeas, beans, broccoli, and dark green leafy vegetables. These foods naturally contain a form of folate that is more bioavailable and generally easier for the body to use.

Methylated versions of supplements like folate (methylfolate) and B-12 (Methylcobalamin, hydroxocobalamin, or adenosylcobalamin) are often recommended, as well as the biologically active form of vitamin B6 (pyridoxal-5-phosphate or P-5-P).

Besides, avoid synthetic folic acid, you also want to avoid the synthetic version of B12 (cyanocobalamin) and instead use the bioactive forms (methylcobalamin, hydroxocobalamin, and adenosylcobalamin).

Avoid exposure to environmental toxins and eat a clean diet wherever possible as the detoxification process is slowed with MTHFR defect.

PureGenomics B-Complex by Pure Encapsulation is my favorite B-complex supplement. It is designed specifically to address the nutrient requirements of common genetic variations in the methylation pathway with a unique blend of bioactive B vitamins. It also contains the optimal doses of methylfolate, methylcobalamin and P5P vitamin B6.

PHASE 3

FEED THE ADHD GUT

It's not just "you are what you eat,"

it's also "you are what you absorb."

Did you know 70% of your body immunity is in the gut?

Healing the leaky ADHD gut is one of the essential steps in the *Eat to Focus Protocol*.

For parents of children with ADHD, you're not going to go wrong getting your children eating a healthy diet in general. A gut-healthy diet involves a variety of foods, including organic meat – organic grass-fed animal protein and wild-caught seafood, colorful, low glycemic index organic produce are ideal.

You want to have diversity in your diet, which also increases the intestinal gut bacteria population's diversity. The more diversified your gut bacteria, the better your overall immunity.

Continue to avoid any artificial food additives and non-GMO foods, as discussed in step 1 Clean Start.

The primary strategy here is to minimize irritation to the gut lining and minimize stimulations of the gut immune system to give the gut a chance to heal and rebalance itself.

Out-of-balance gut causes problems for everyone. Kids with ADHD seem to already have a weak immune system that causes allergies and low-grade inflammation in the brain, resulting in ADHD symptoms.

Children with ADHD can't get away with treating the gut bacteria the way that many other people do.

Signs that Your Child's Gut Flora is Imbalanced
There are numerous clinical signs of imbalanced bowel flora. And here are the more common red flags:

- Abnormal bowel patterns, such as frequent diarrhea, chronic constipation, poorly digested food in stool regularly, frequent unusual stool color or odor, or onset of urine or stool incontinence in previously potty-trained children.

- Explosive behaviors, such as tantrums, extreme irritability, sensory irritability, especially for noise, or silliness or hyperactivity following a starchy meal.

- Physical symptoms include ringworm rash, intermittent diffuse rashes of unknown origin, acne, history of oral thrush, persisting diaper rash, or bloated belly.

- Frequent use of antibiotics disrupts the normal gut balance between healthy bugs in the gut (Lactobacillus, bifidobacteria, e. Coli) and other potentially dangerous bugs, including yeasts, bacteria, and occasionally parasites.

Symptoms of yeast or candida overgrowth are very similar to those of other conditions, but you are more likely to have a yeast problem if you have any of these conditions.

- Oral thrush
- Bloatedness and gassiness
- Intestinal cramp
- Rectal itching
- constipation or diarrhea
- Fatigue or lack of energy
- Intense cravings for sugar and refined carbohydrates
- Skin and nail fungal infections, such as athlete's foot or toenail fungus

How to Correct Gut Microbiome Imbalance?

1. Correct Digestion

If you have been following the Phase 1 and Phase 2 of the *Eat to Focus Protocol* in eliminating all the food on the list and replenish with brain-nourishing food, you should have seen some improvement in digestion already.

But we want better than just some improvement, so here we go.

- Eat slowly and chew food thoroughly. Remember, your parents used to tell you to slow down and chew your food well. And your parents are right.

    Digestion starts in the mouth. Try to maximize digestion by being relaxed while eating, taking small bites, and thoroughly chewing your food.

    Chewing your food well helps to **nourish your gut with salivary Epidermal Growth Factor (EGF)**, which is found in high concentrations in salivary glands and the duodenum. EGF is a polypeptide that stimulates the growth and repair of epithelial tissue of the intestine.

- Take one tablespoon of lemon juice or apple cider vinegar mixed with water with meals. Our stomach makes stomach acid that kills incoming bacteria and helps to break down protein. Many people do not make enough stomach acid, causing poor digestion of protein and bacteria setting camp in the stomach and intestines.

  Adding lemon juice or apple cider vinegar during meals will help increase the stomach's acidity to break down protein more efficiently in the stomach and improve protein absorption in the small intestines.

- Take digestive enzymes to help break down food properly and increase nutrient absorption. Our body makes special enzymes to break down carbohydrates, protein, and fats in the small intestines.

  Sometimes our body needs a little extra help to properly breaking down the food. If food is not adequately broken down, then partially digested food can enter the bloodstream through the leaky gut and trigger allergic reactions, which may worsen ADHD symptoms.

Pure Encapsulation Digestive Enzymes Ultra is what I recommend the most. The capsules are small and easy to swallow. And it contains a variety of enzymes, not just the standard amylase, lipase, and protease.

2. Patch up the leaky gut

- Glycine-rich food, such as bone broth, organs, connective tissue, helps repair leaky gut and minimize allergic food reactions.
- Collagen is beneficial to gut health because it contains large amounts of the amino acids glycine, glutamine and proline which can be beneficial to the intestinal tract as well as the stomach. Collagen as a foundational building block, providing strength and structure for our connective tissues.
- Glutamine supplements are beneficial as well for gut health. Glutamine is an essential substrate for the maintenance of intestinal metabolism and integrity. *Glutamine supplementation has been shown to reverse intestinal mucosal injury, resulting in less villous atrophy, increased mucosal healing, and decreased endotoxin passage through the gut wall.*

- Take a daily zinc supplement, especially if your child always complains that food tastes or smells funny and has diarrhea. Zinc helps with healing the leaky gut while also boost the immune system. Oral zinc supplements can reduce the symptoms of diarrhea in children with low levels of zinc. I like using zinc carnosine. It helps protect the stomach and intestinal lining and helps with heartburn or gastroesophageal reflux. I personally use **Integrative Therapeutics Zinc Carnosine**, which is chelated zinc, meaning easier to absorb.
- Vitamin C supplements to support healing.
- Avoid dairy, gluten, grains, and legumes. Refer to Step 1 Clean Start.
- Avoid chronic medication use with antibiotics, antacids, and steroids, which can disrupt the gut permeability.
- Avoid NSAIDS pain-killers. They are known to cause intestinal bleeding.

3. Correct Gut Microbiome

Correcting intestinal flora is an essential and critical step for helping a child who has learning, behavior, or developmental challenges be happier and healthier. There are also studies showing that probiotic supplements help improve depressive symptoms, anger, and fatigue in children with ADHD.

Probiotics Supplements

Probiotics supplements are the first tool to correct gut microbiome. This is especially important if your child is born via c-section and bottle-fed the first year. Both of these events prevented your child from acquiring the beneficial gut flora from the birth canal and breastmilk.

Taking a probiotic supplement is an excellent way to add more good bacteria to your intestines. This will also help crowd out the harmful bacteria.

Many years ago, I had a patient who had 32 bunnies living in their 2-bedroom house. They're family of 4. The rabbits took up one room, and the whole family sleeps in the other bedroom. I asked them why they have so many bunnies. The parents said they started with only two rabbits, and next thing you know, they have almost three dozen bunnies.

You may or may not need the maintenance after everything is corrected. Probiotics are also like goldfish. You don't keep buying new goldfish in your tank once you have enough, right?

When you start probiotics and give your bacteria a nice comfortable home, the bacteria will thrive and multiple like these bunnies.

Chewable probiotic tablets and eating yogurt daily is not useful for correcting imbalances. These are okay for daily maintenance.

Besides, many special needs children have casein intolerance and therefore, cannot eat yogurt made with dairy products, so appropriate supplementation becomes more important.

Bifidobacteria with a little Lactobacillus is an excellent blend for babies up to a year old.

Toddlers can shift to blends that emphasize Lactobacillus and other strains.

Older children who have gut dysbiosis need higher potencies of probiotic, starting in the range of 50 billion "colony forming units" (CFUs) per dose once a day plus a high dose beneficial yeast supplement, such as one capsule once a day.

How much probiotics do you need?

- To correct gut microbiome imbalance: 50 billion CFU's x1-2 times per day 30 min after meals. Take _Vitamin Bounty Pro 50 Probiotic with Prebiotics - 13 Strains, 50 Billion CFU_ one capsule 30 minutes after each meal.

- To correct yeast overgrowth: In addition to a high dose probiotics, add 5 billion CFUs saccharomyces boulardii (beneficial yeast) daily. Take _Jarrow Formulas Saccharomyces Boulardii + MOS, 5 Billion CFU_ one cap daily.

- Maintenance dose if needed: 1 cap of 10-20 billion BID 30mins after each meal. The _Lovebug Probiotic and Prebiotic for Kids_ (15 Billion CFU) is the only decent kids' probiotics on the market. All the other kids' probiotics only have a pathetic 3 billion CFUs per dose.

Fermented Foods and Beverages

Eat fermented foods and beverages such as coconut milk kefir, kombucha, kimchee, raw sauerkraut, and coconut yogurt are packed with probiotics. Eat at least one of these daily. Choose only low-sugar, guar-gum-free coconut yogurt, especially if they are homemade or obtained from local sources.

Remember, taking the probiotics supplement is not enough. You need to feed your "pet" (probiotics) with a high fiber diet. Otherwise, they'll keep dying off of hunger and starvation. And you'll be wasting your probiotic supplements.

We all know kitty eats cat food. And doggie eats dog food.

Since we know the good and bad guys eat a different diet. We're going to feed more of the clean eating we discussed in Step 2 that the good bacteria prefers, and restrict the bad guys' diet of junk food.

When this happens, the harmful bacteria will soon die because of a lack of food for them. And the good bacteria will continue to flourish on the clean eating diet and less environmental competition from the harmful bacteria.

Anti-fungal Supplements

Natural anti-fungal supplements can also help get rid of yeast and candida faster. These are naturally occurring compounds that can be very helpful in controlling yeast. These include grapefruit seed extract, olive leaf extract, calendula, oregano oil, goldenseal, garlic, tea tree, black walnut, pau d'arco, cranberry extract, and caprylic acid (from coconut oil).

Remove Sugar from Diet

When you remove sugar from your diet, you're also removing the food that bacteria and yeast thrive on —eliminating sugar in all of its simple forms, such as candy, desserts, alcohol, wheat flours, complex whole-grain carbohydrates, like grains, beans, fruit, bread, pasta, and potatoes.

Replace high sugar food with high fiber low glycemic index food. Use stevia or monk fruit as sugar alternatives. The yeast and bad bacteria will starve and eventually die.

Avoid Antibiotics

Antibiotics kill both good and bad bacteria. But if you really need the antibiotics for a nasty infection, make sure to eat some fermented food and take a probiotics supplement. Be sure to take the probiotics and antibiotics at least 2 hours apart from each other.

Relax and Breathe.

Stress can be a massive contributor to a leaky gut and gut imbalance. Activities that promote relaxation and lower stress hormones also help heal the leaky gut. Activities such as yoga, meditation, walk in nature, hiking, exercise, etc., not only reduce your stress hormones, but they also increase your feel-good hormone – endorphins.

Follow these steps for at least 2-3 months to see improvements. That's how long it takes for the intestine to rebalance itself.

PHASE 4

BRAIN REBOOT

"Rome wasn't built in one day…"

Treating ADHD naturally it's not all about just food and vitamins. Things you do to take care of your body are just as important.

Food and nutrition correct any food intolerance that's causing trouble while bringing in the building blocks and signals to the game, but your body has to do its job to put everything in the right place.

And this is what **Phase 4 Brain Reboot** is all about - putting things in the right place.

In Phase 4 Brain Reboot, you'll learn what strategies to get your child the necessary sleep they need for healing, and what exercises are best for the mind and body to increase calm and focus.

The brain is a organ that uses a lot of energy, and it acts just like a muscle. The more you use it, the fitter and more efficient your brain would be. On the other hand, too much reliance on technology and lack of challenge cause the brain to become flabby or slow.

When I daughter was 8 years old, she fell off the monkey bar on the first day at school. She broke her wrist and had to be in a cast for 6 weeks. When the cast finally came off, her left arm become significantly skinnier than her right arm because of lack of use for 6 weeks.

Fortunately, young children recovers quickly. She quickly regained all functions and strength of her left arm in no time.

The brain atrophies just like the arm in a cast for month, the brain connection becomes weak and slow.

Fortunately, the human brain is magical and completely able to heal and rebuild.

Scientists used to believe that the human brain stopped growing by late adolescence, after which our brain would never change or grow further, other than to deteriorate.

We now know that's not true.

Scientists now discovered that the human brain is always changing and molding itself to your surroundings and challenges you put it through. Our brains can change and be shaped by our actions and environment.

Because our brains are subject to our genes, actions and environment, we each have our very own unique brain to us. Our brains are like snowflakes. There are no two identical brains. Each brain adapts to the needs of its owner.

Every time your brain learns something new, it creates a new synaptic connection. Every time this happens, your brain physically changes to upgrade its hardware to reflect a new mind level.

The more you repeat or practice the same action, the stronger and faster the connections become.

The human brain has an incredible ability to change its structure and rewire over time by forming new nerve cell connections as we experience or adapt to new challenges.

One of these examples is people, who suffer from strokes, recover and regain their brain function and body functions again.

A group of researchers at the University College of London studied the London taxi driver to look at how memorizing such a disorganized street system has on the brain.

Why London taxi driver?

In London, earning the license to drive one of the city's iconic cabs is equivalent to earning a university degree. Earning the taxi driver's license in London is mused to be equivalent to getting a black belt in karate while becoming an Eagle Scout while vying for admission to Mensa.

The knowledge required to earn the license is so advanced that being able to navigate the streets isn't just considered knowledge but is formally called "The Knowledge."

The 'Knowledge,' as it is known, provides a lovely real-world example of expertise. But unlike most other examples of expertise development (e.g., music, chess, sports, arts), it is mostly unaffected by childhood experience.

It is developed through a training program over a short period of time common to all participants. And these participants are of average IQ (average verbal IQ was around or just below 100) and average education (average school-leaving age was around 16.7 years) for all groups.

The part of the brain that navigates spatial intelligence is called the hippocampus, a pair of two chestnut-sized masses toward the back of your head. The researchers found that licensed London taxi drivers have a uniquely bigger hippocampi than almost anyone else.

So what underlies this development of the posterior hippocampus?

If the qualified and non-qualified trainees were comparable in education and IQ, what determined whether a trainee would 'build-up' his hippocampus and pass the exams?

The obvious answer is hard work and dedication, and this is borne out by the fact that, although the two groups were similar in the length of their training period, those who qualified spent significantly more time training every week (an average of 34.5 hours a week vs. 16.7 hours). Those who qualified also attended far more tests (an average of 15.6 vs. 2.6).

This study shows directly and within individuals how the structure of the hippocampus can change with external stimulation and that the human brain remains 'plastic' even into adulthood, allowing it to adapt when we need to learn new tasks.

Brain Gym

Exercise benefits your brain in more ways than you can imagine. Research after research has shown that physical activities can benefit children and adolescents with ADHD.

Exercise improves motor skills, physical fitness, attention, and social behaviors in children with ADHD. Neuroscientists show that a single workout will immediately increase brain chemicals, such as dopamine, serotonin, and noradrenaline, to improve your ability to focus up to at least 2 hours after exercise.

Long-term exercise improves attention, and the volume of the hippocampus and prefrontal cortex increases as well. Exercise also has a protective effect on the brain.

Remember the brain is like a muscle. The more you work out, the bigger and stronger the hippocampus and prefrontal cortex get, and the longer before age-related degenerative brain disorders hit.

This is important because the hippocampus and prefrontal cortex are two areas most susceptible to neurodegenerative disease and age-related cognitive decline.

There is also a large body of research on the beneficial effects of exercise on depression and anxiety. The results of exercise as a treatment for mild to moderate depression compare favorably to psychotherapy and pharmacologic treatment.

Exercise not only helps to reduce stress, but it also helps to reduce fatigue, improve mood, alertness, concentration, and overall cognitive function.

The rule of thumb is 30 minutes of cardio activities x3-4 times a week.

Detox with Exercise

The human body has two circulatory systems – the first one is where blood circulates, the other is the lymphatic system.

The heart is involved in moving blood throughout the body into and out of all organs, like a transportation system carrying vital nutrients to all parts of the body.

The lymphatic circulation is more like a "police patrol" system going around the body looking for "criminals" to arrest. The lymphatic system is our detox or criminal justice system.

The lymphatic circulation does not have an assistance like the heart to help with blood circulation. The only way to keep this system flowing is by moving. The movement of muscle contributes to the stimulation circulation of the lymphatic fluid through the lymphatic ducts. Massage and yoga are other ways to keep the lymphatic ducts moving.

Anti-Inflammatory Effect of Exercise

While chronic stress stokes the fire in the inflammatory response, acute stress but controlled stress can have just the opposite effect, essentially the opposite of chronic stress, thereby lessening inflammation.

Resistance or strength training is one of the best ways to put your body in a state of acute but controlled stress.

A review of research on the anti-inflammatory effects of exercise found that resistance training can play a significant role in reducing cytokines' circulating levels, the body's inflammation signals.

For example, in one study, researchers found that women who followed a moderately high resistance training program for 24-weeks had lower levels of circulating cortisol.

Participants were instructed to lift weights four times a week, progressing to more challenging exercises and alternating between endurance (high reps for 2-3 sets) and strength (1-6 reps repeated for four sets).

Similarly, decreased circulating cortisol levels were reported after just 8-weeks of resistance training that encompassed a full-body workout.

Based on this evidence, the best exercise plan is 30 minutes of cardio exercise x3-4 times a week and 30 minutes of resistance training x4 times a week. The best time to exercise is in the morning to reap the mental focus and energy boost during work or school. But if evening works best for you, still do it.

Let's Get Physical…

You don't need to join the gym or sign-up for Cross Fit to get the benefits of exercise.

Just put on some comfortable shoes and go for a power walk or jog for 30 minutes. This will be your cardio. Then 30 minutes of yoga for resistance training. You can pull up *yoga for beginners* video easily from youtube.com.

To help get into the mindset of daily physical activities, I often ask my patients to start every morning with ten jumping jacks. This way, you get a sense of accomplishment and hopefully continue to stay on track. Doing ten jumping jacks is so easy, there's almost no excuse not to do it. This gets you into the daily activity mentality. And get the blood flowing.

This will take care of the problem most people frequently have, "I don't have time," "I'm tired." When you are doing just this simple ten jumping jacks a day, you start feeling good about yourself and want to do more. And before you know it, you've just created a new exercise habit, and you may be doing more than just jumping jacks then.

When I first started running more than ten years ago, I can only run for about a minute or so. Then I had to stop, caught up with my breath, and began again. That did not stop me. I keep running and stopping. And you know what, since then I'd run multiple short races, half marathons, marathons, and triathlons.

I'm not going to lie to you. It's going to be tough in the beginning finding the motivation. That's why I ask you to only start with ten jumping jacks. If you can't even do this, then no one else can help you.

Start asking yourself "why" you want to make this lifestyle change. Focus on the brain and emotional benefits of exercise. Focus on the joy you'll have spending quality time with your happy, healthy child who does not need ADHD medication to focus.

Again, you need to do it with your child. Make it fun. As long as something is fun, your child will do it. Give your child a sense of control, let him or her pick the exercise to do for the day - jumping jacks, squats, lunges, crunches or planks.

If possible, do these in the morning as the brain benefit of exercise with help your child during school.

Keep track of your progress. Studies have shown that people who track their fitness progress tend to have better results and continue with the new lifestyle changes.

I use the SweatCoin app to keep track of my daily steps and earn SweatCoins while doing it.

In Hawaii, it's easy to stay active all year long. During the week, I work out at the gym, and on weekends, we go hiking, stand-up paddling, playing tennis, playing golf, etc.

Find something that the whole family can enjoy together and convenient to do every day.

Yoga

How could we talk about meditation, and not talk about yoga? They are always practiced together.

Parents often think that kids need to be out running around to let out of energy, but staying inside doing some calming exercise such as yoga is beneficial.

Before I started practicing yoga, *I used to think yoga is so easy*. I always see yoga people doing these simple poses, no sweating, like eating a piece of cake. And I thought how hard can that be?

Then, I took my first yoga class. Boy...*I was wrong about yoga.*

Yoga is not easy, but not hard either. It's just challenging, and I love challenges.

After each yoga class, *my body would hurt in places that I did not know exists before*. But I love the feeling of "good hurt," which comes with a sense of accomplishment and freedom.

Yoga is an excellent exercise for anyone, especially kids with ADHD because it provides *a full-body stimulation experience*. Practicing *yoga can increase calming chemicals in the brain and strengthen the prefrontal cortex*, which helps reduce symptoms of depression, anxiety, and even seizures.

Here are 3 Benefits of Yoga for Kids with ADHD

1. Yoga Increases Focus & Concentration

When kids concentrate on their breath or feel a stretch in their arms, *they learn body awareness*. This teaches them to keep their minds in one place instead of all over the place.

One study found that children who *practiced yoga for just 20 minutes two times a week for eight weeks had better scores on tests that measure attention and focus*.

The *self-control eventually spills over to the classroom and home*. You'll start to notice you're not yelling as often. Homework time becomes less stressful. You begin getting sweet notes from teachers and principles from school.

You may still find a moldy sandwich in their backpacks here and there. Some kids are just messy.

2. Yoga Increases Calmness

Yoga also includes some breathing technique that I talked about for meditation. *Part of yoga is to focus on breathing and what the body is doing.*

Most of us do not breathe properly or enough. And we tend to take shallow breaths from our chest, rather than breathing fully from our diaphragm—which gives you a deep, cleansing breath.

Breathing slowly and deeply through the nose is a powerful tool to reduce day-to-day stress and calm the mind down.

Another study showed that *practicing yoga for 60 minutes, three times a week for 12 weeks, shows considerable improvements in mood and anxiety* than just walking alone.

3. Yoga Increases Confidence

Yoga not only helps with calming and focus but, most of all, confidence. *Having ADHD takes a lot of confidence away from your child.* Yoga helps to build confidence by trying new activities and developing new skills.

When they practice the same poses and become good at it, it gives them the confidence to keep going. Kids learn self-control and self-calming techniques, which helps to improve their social skills.

I have included five fun yoga poses for you and your new yogi to practice.

Once your child gets confident with these, then help them find new poses to try. ***Practice the postures in the same order every time for consistency and build memory muscles.***

Another great thing about yoga is that you can do it anywhere.

Ready to start?

Here are a few kid-friendly yoga moves that you and your family can do right now.

It's easy to make yoga fun because initially, all the yoga moves feel silly. So just have fun, don't worry if you're doing it with perfect form.

Holding a yoga pose can be difficult, both mentally and physically, for kids with ADHD. So when they complete a pose successfully, celebrate the little victories with them.

A Fun Shape-Shifting Yoga Sequence for Kids

1. Mountain Pose: Stand up straight with feet together, touching and arms on the side. Spread the toes and straighten the legs without locking the knees. Stand as tall as possible by pushing both feet on the ground while lifting through the head, making sure to face forward and keeping your head level. Hold for ten deep breaths.

2. Tree Pose: Transition from the Mountain Pose to Tree Pose to hide from your parents. Start with lifting one leg and resting the foot on the inside of the standing leg. You may use to hands to move your leg. Then, put your hands together into a prayer gesture. Now you know being a tree is not easy. Try to hold for ten deep breaths, then repeat for the other leg.

3. Downward Dog or Down Dog Pose: Now transition from the Tree Pose to the Down Dog Pose. The Tree is tired of being peed on all the time. Put your leg down from the tree pose, then bend forward until your hands touch the ground and walk your hands slowly forward until your body forms a triangle with the ground. Hold for ten deep breaths again.

4. Sphinx Pose: From the Down Dog, you shapeshift into the Sphinx pose. Drop your knees to the ground and walk your hands forward until you're on your belly. Then lift your upper body and rest on your elbows, just like the Great

Sphinx in Egypt. Hold for ten deep breaths.

5. **Child's Pose:** Now, you're going back into a human child. Scoot your body up on all fours and walk your hands backward until your butt is sitting on your legs. Then lean forward with your arms stretched above your head on the ground while keeping your butt down. I don't know how to explain it. If you get confused, look at the pictures. Hold for ten deep breaths.

Schedule some yoga time every day. You'll be surprised what it can do for your child and your family.

Quiet Time Quiet Mind

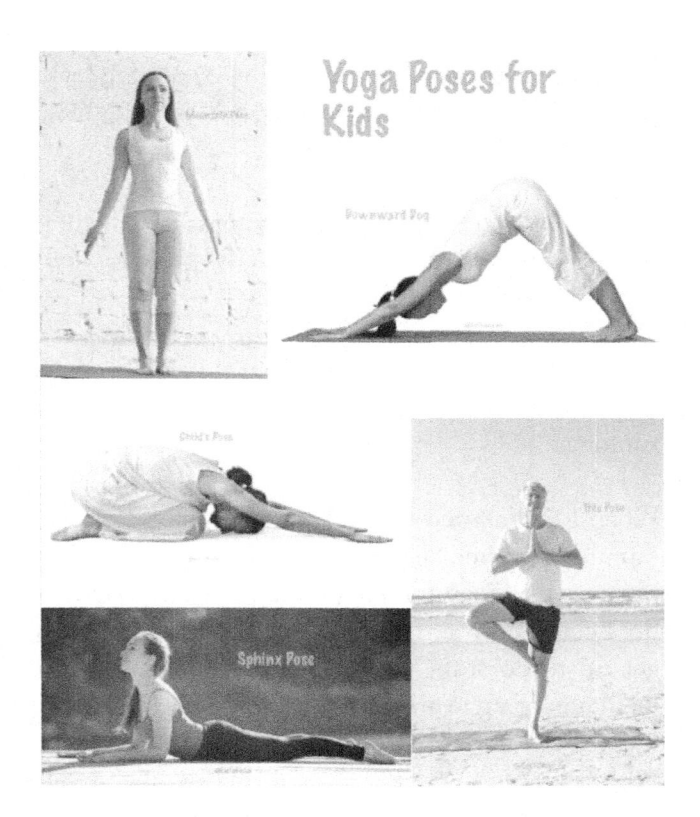

I can see your eyes rolling, reading the title.

You've probably seen pictures of people meditating sitting still for an extended period of time, and you're like, "my child will never be able to do that."

Not so quick to judge…

Meditation is a very calming and refreshing experience. The practice of meditation involves a lot of focus and concentration. And focus and concentration are what many children with ADHD are lacking. But, it does not mean meditation is impossible for children with ADHD.

Everything you read about mindfulness and meditation sounds so deep - self-awareness, presence, and all that.

I don't get all of those either, but what I know is meditation is a skill that anyone can get at just like running.

When I first started meditation, I can only do a few minutes at a time because I constantly want to open my eyes as I keep thinking of all the tasks I have to do. I could only sit for a few minutes, and I need to get up to do stuff. I keep practicing. Today, I can meditate for up to an hour.

With "practice," I'm able to "still" my monkey brain and meditate for more extended periods.

So meditation is a practice that you build up on. For the beginner, maybe have your child lie down on the floor or bed for a few minutes.

You may look at meditation as a form of "brain yoga" that changes your mind's level of consciousness by bringing your mind inward into your inner self. For starter, 5 minutes a day is good.

You see people meditating, and it looks so easy… you just sit cross-legged with eyes closed.

Once I got the hang of it, I enjoy meditation. It feels like doing yoga for the brain because you're trying to wrestle your mind to a still position where you start having "mystical images." This is where you achieve the alpha brain waves. It's the calm brain waves right before you drift off to sleep, but not quite asleep.

Whatever that means…it means shutting down the outside and stay inside if you understand what I mean.

To me, being in a meditative state is like being in my own "Anna's in the Wonderland." You're in between awake and asleep.

It's abstract…you have to try it to understand. But it takes practice to get there.

The fascinating thing about meditation is that it can change brain waves and brain activities. Researches and studies have shown structural and physiological changes in the brain with frequent meditation.

It has many physiological benefits, and increasing focus and concentration are a few. Thousands of researches and studies have shown the benefits of meditation and its effects on metabolism, blood pressure, brain activation, and other bodily processes.

When we first started meditation, my daughter did not like it. Just the thought of sitting down and doing nothing for 5 minutes sounds like torture to her. She was ten years old, so it is still quite easy to persuade her to do it.
She would set her own timer on her watch, which gives her some feeling of control. We try to do it every day, but of course, it's hit or miss.

After meditating several times, my daughter did acknowledge some benefits, such as feeling calm, refreshed, and increased alertness, which helped clear her mind for mentally demanding tasks. Now she does not fight me as much if I ask her to meditate before starting her homework. Yet, 5 minutes is still what she is up for.

For starter, aim for five minutes or less, something that you know your child can comfortably handle. Be sure to make it fun. Otherwise, they are not going to do it again.

I used to snuggle with my daughter in her bed at bedtime. Then I would let her put one of her favorite stuffed animals on her belly while lying on her back. I would ask her to take deep breaths until she sees her stuffed animal rises and falls on her belly.

This helps to teach her the breathing part of the practice. The trick is taking long deep breaths that fill up the belly. Slowly you can add the counting from 1-10 to make the breaths longer.

Think of it as "quiet time." Even if your child can't sit with their eyes close for 5 minutes, have them start by being quiet for 5 minutes, not making any noise or big movements.

They can play with their stuffed animals, draw, or whatever they want. You can also play some soothing music in the background. This quiet time can also be used as a transition to the next tasks or activities.

You can also do the "quiet time" right before bed. Snuggle with your child, read a story, and kiss him or her good night. Then turn off the lights. Some children have difficulty falling asleep.

Be firm and tell your child, so he or she knows that he or she has to stay in the dark room and not make noise. A small night light is allowed. Most children will eventually fall asleep.

Adding the "om" is beneficial as well. The vibration of the "Om" chant, believe it or not, massages the vagus nerve, calms the nervous system.

Research shows that mindfulness training improves attention span and helps with self-regulation, which is missing in individuals with ADHD.

Countries in Southeast Asia has been practicing meditation for over two thousand years. It has always been associated with religious rituals. However, it has no religious boundaries. Anyone can practice this mental art form, regardless of faith or belief.

Mindfulness and yoga are commonly practiced in the general community to improve mental and physical health. Parents, teachers, and healthcare providers are also increasingly using such interventions with children.

Learning to Breath

The practice of mediation teaches you to focus on your breathing and learn to breathe correctly. While we all breathe without thinking, most of us do not breathe properly or enough.

Most of us tend to breathe from our chest, shallow breaths, rather than breathing fully from our diaphragm—which gives you an in-depth, cleansing breath.

Breathing slowly and deeply through the nose is a powerful tool to decrease your day-to-day stress.

Breathing through the nose can help to reduce stress by stimulating the parasympathetic nervous system.

When we start taking nice long deep breaths, the extra oxygen gives our bodies a big boost of oxygen, our body is craving.

It increases your sense of well-being, increased energy levels (the right kind), reduced anxiety, and reduced irritability.

Learning how to breathe correctly can help children feel more in control of their brains and bodies, which is huge for a kid with ADHD.

Music to the Brain

Music can be a fun, therapeutic activity for your child. Music therapy can improve focus and attention, reduce hyperactivity, and improve social skills.

When my daughter was eight years old, we enrolled her in piano lessons hoping that it would calm her down and help her sit still.

Well, it did. She loves music and loves playing the piano. But she hated to practice. She does not play much piano now because I pushed her too hard with practice.

Nonetheless, she still loves music. And she's kind of a music snob.

When I meditate or work, I like to play soothing spa music in the background to help ease my mind into stillness or emptiness.

My daughter called it "depressing music." I call it "brain massage" music. I like to listen to meditation music while I'm working or mediating when I need to concentrate and not get distracted by the surrounding noise. The spa music helps me to stay in the *focus zone*.

Without music, I feel like my brain has holes where all my attention is leaking out. The music helps to fill those holes and keep my attention inside and stay focus.

The long and slow melody feels like long massage strokes going through my brain.

I especially like the piano and harp music. Each strum of the note feels like a tension spot is released in my brain.

Put on some "brain massage" music sit quietly in a comfortable space and just enjoy the music and relax your brain.

Search for relaxing music for study on youtube.com and play it in the background while your child is doing homework or studying.

In my experience, I feel the music works better listened to in a headphone.

My daughter just returned from Chicago after her first semester of freshman year. She told me that music from *the Phantom of the Opera* is the best music for her homework and studying.

So experiment with different genres of music and see which one works best for your child. Generally, you want to stick with just melody for homework. I avoid music with words because sometimes I get my writing and thinking confused with lyrics from the songs.

Healing Hours

Sleep is when all the growing and healing happen. Have you ever notice that children tend to grow significantly in length over the summer break? Is it coincidence, or is it because they're sleeping more during summer?

We are always told, "you need to sleep 8 to be great!"

So why do we need 8 hours of sleep a night?

Recently I went to a conference called *"Pharmacy in the Kitchen"* by Dr. Micheal Lara, M.D.

And it is during this conference that I learned about the reason why we need to sleep for eight full hours. Not just for us adults, but more importantly, our kids.

There are four stages of sleep, as shown in the picture above. Most of us go through all the stages of sleep. These stages progress cyclically from stage 1 through stage 4, Rapid-Eye-Movement (REM) sleep, then start the next cycle at stage 1 again. A complete sleep cycle takes an average of 90 to 110 minutes, with each stage lasting between 5 to 15 minutes.

The first couple of sleep cycles each night have relatively short REM sleeps and longer periods of deep sleep (stage 3 and 4), but later in the night, REM sleep periods lengthen and deep sleep time decreases.

During the first half of the 8-hour sleep cycle, our body is in the deepest sleep (stage 3 & 4). This is where our body does all the repairs and recovery from the damages sustained throughout the day. This is where children grow. It is also this deep sleep stages that provide the anti-inflammatory benefits of sleep.

Okay, this is the first 4 hours.

Then, the second half of your sleep cycle is just as important. Instead of having a deeper sleep, your body is now experiencing longer and longer REM cycle sleep as the night progresses.

The REM sleep cycle is when your brain consolidates your short-term memories accumulated during the day into long-term memory.

Kids, this is why you need to go to bed early and get full 8 hours of sleep every night, so you can grow taller, learn faster, and build better memories.

Everything you learn and experience during the day will become a permanent memory in an 8-hour sleep cycle.

So don't miss out.

How Many Hours of Sleep Should Your Kiddo Have Every Night?

Children need their sleep. There are no excuses.

- **Babies**: 11-17 hours per day (0-3 months old) and 12-15 hours per day (4-11 months old)
- **Toddlers**: 11-14 hours per day (1-2 years old)
- **Preschool**: 10-13 hours per day (3-5 years old)
- **School-age**: 9-11 hours per day (6-13 years old)
- **Teenage**: 8-10 hours per day (14-17 years old)

Sleep disorders are common in children with ADHD. Initially, everyone thought it was side effects of ADHD medication. Studies later showed that 30-40 percent of children with ADHD have sleep disorders, whether they are taking medication or not.

As we learned so far, people with ADHD have abnormal metabolism of brain chemicals, which makes sense that their bodies do not produce enough melatonin at night.

Chronic stress can also affect the production and secretion of the hormone. Stress could be from both physical and mental sources, and even metabolic stress from the environment.

Common sleep disorders in kids with ADHD are restless legs syndrome, obstructive sleep apnea, snoring, sleepwalking, and night terrors.

Although people with ADHD notoriously have difficulty sleeping, they may or may not have a sleep disorder. The inability to get a good night's sleep interferes with many daytime activities.

When you don't get enough sleep, you can have a hard time focusing, communicating, following directions, and may even suffer decreased short-term memory. People with ADHD may experience many of these symptoms, unrelated to getting a good night's sleep.

Bedtime is often another battle beside dinner. Every night without fail, my daughter would be hungry when it's time for bed. You know how you always give in when your child says, "I'm hungry"?

Especially, my daughter, who rarely eats, so when she says she's hungry, you just willing to comply. I was such a sucker for that. It's her tricks to stay up later.

Did you know it's also very important that your child goes to bed at the same time every night, whether it's weekdays or weekends?

I know it is a lot easier just to let the weekend go and let your kids sleep whenever they want, one less battle to fight.

Unfortunately, an inconsistent bedtime routine can be a considerable drawback.

A United Kingdom study looked at the bedtime habits of 10,000 kids between 3 and 7 years old and found that kids with inconsistent bedtimes had more behavioral difficulties than those with consistent bedtime routines.

The researchers found that kids who did not go to bed at the same time every night scored higher on unhappiness, being inconsiderate, and fighting.

Those scores came not only from parent reports but also from teachers, who rated the kids without regular bedtimes to have more problematic behaviors.

Going to bed at 8 o'clock one night and 10 o'clock the next can create some kind of "jet lag," even if they're getting the same hours of sleep.

It's like jet lag from flying through different time zones, your child's body gets shuffled through different time zones, and their circadian rhythms and hormonal systems take a hit.

The good news is that these negative effects on behavior are reversible.

When kids in the study switched from having irregular bedtimes to a regular bedtime, there were measurable improvements in their behavior.

This shows that it's never too late to help children back onto a positive path, and a small change could make a big difference in how well they get on.

In a follow-up study published in 2017, the researchers also found that irregular bedtimes don't just impact behaviors, but can also put kids at risk for obesity and low-self esteem, and tank their math scores.

Regular bedtimes can have a positive impact on a kid's development, health, and behavior.

So the next time you're tempted to let bedtime slide, remember that by being strict with bedtime, you're not only protecting your sleep and self-care time but also protecting your child's circadian rhythms and mental health.

Start with a calming bedtime routine to help your child wind down. Turn lights down low. Limit loud noises and bright lights, such as from electronics. Read a real paper book and even meditate to relax the mind.

Some of you may have noticed that your child has started sleeping better since starting the *Eat to Focus Program*. And here are four more natural remedies you can try if you still need help in this area.

4 Natural Remedies to Help You Get Your Child to Sleep Without a Fight

1. Foot Massage

I used to massage my daughter's feet to get her to fall asleep. Whenever I get foot massage during massages, I always fall asleep, so I figured there must be something relaxing with massaging the feet.

Foot massage or sometimes referred to as reflexology is an ancient technique used to change your body's energies. According to the study of reflexology, stimulating different pressure points on the feet, you can subtly impact the glands and organs around your entire body.

It helps people with sleep issues by calming the nervous system, promoting relaxation, and reducing stress and pain.

Studies in China and Korea showed that reflexology helps with relaxation by inducing the alpha and theta waves. Researchers also saw a decrease in blood pressure and anxiety.

Alpha waves help with overall mental coordination, calmness, alertness, mind/body connection, and learning.

Theta brainwaves occur most often in sleep and deep meditation. Theta is our gateway to learning, memory, and intuition.

Now get a foot massage...

2. Epsom Salt

Epsom salt is said to have been discovered in the late middle ages when a farmer in Epsom, England, noticed the *water flowing through his property soothed skin wounds.*

Water from the Epsom's springs is infused with *magnesium sulfate, which helps ease muscle aches and pains, exfoliate dead skin cells, soothe sore feet, improve sleep, and reduce stress.*

Epsom salt's main component is magnesium sulfate ($MgSO_4$). It is harvested from the springs that arise where the North Downs' porous chalk meets non-porous London clay. It is named after an English town, "Epsom" in Surrey, England, from which this salt originates.

Epsom salt is *traditionally used as a bath salt* for relieving muscle aches/pains, insect bug bites, sunburns, replenishing youthful skin, and detoxification.

People often think the *toxins inside the body are being drawn from the skin pores into the bathwater*. The truth is that soaking in the Epsom salt bath allows the body to absorb the magnesium and sulfate through the skin into the body. Then *the body gets rid of toxin via its detoxification system*.

The secret is in the sulfate. The Epsom salt provides the *sulfate needed in the detoxification process in the liver*. This *influx of sulfate boosts the liver's detoxification system*, and toxins are then released via the colon or kidneys.

How to Use Epsom Salt to Help Your ADHD Child Calm Down?

You can do an *Epsom salt bath or foot soak or paste*.

Epsom Salt Bath

An Epsom salt bath at night before bed is very relaxing. The warmth of the water and Epsom salt bath can help calm the body.

Simply fill a bathtub with hot water and add 2 cups of Epsom salt. You may also add 1 cup of baking soda and some lavender oil for additional soothing effects. Soak for about 20 minutes.

You may read to your child during this time. Be sure not to leave little children unattended in the bathtub filled with water.

Besides a full bath, you can also do a *foot bath for 15 minutes while doing homework or reading*. Of course, you'll save a lot of water and use a lot less salt.

Epsom Salt Foot Soak

Simply fill up a bucket with hot water and add about 1/4 to 1/2 cup of Epsom salt. You can also add baking soda and any essential oil, just like a bath.

Epsom Salt Paste

I make a *topical paste* that also works wonderfully. It saves time, energy, and water.

For the topical paste, simply dissolve about one teaspoon of the salt with about one teaspoon of water enough to dissolve most of the salt. As the salt dissolves, you'll notice the water thickens slightly. It's okay if not all the salt is dissolved. It just means that solution is saturated with Epsom salt.

Now you can apply this solution onto the skin with a make-up brush or cotton balls. I usually do this on my daughter's legs right before she goes to bed.

You will notice a thin layer of white salt on the skin as the water evaporates. The salt will continue to be absorbed as long as it stays in contact with the skin. You can leave that on because the salt usually gets rubbed off during the night. The sulfate is thought to circulate in the body up to about nine hours.

These are ***best performed before bedtime at night to calm down***.

I have a parent who told me that the Epsom salt makes his son sleepy. This is because magnesium helps calm the brain. Remember, from Phase 2?

Best of all, my daughter stops having that funny smell when she sweats.

Some children may become agitated after taking the Epsom salt bath. If that's the case, ***start the bath with 1/4 cup of Epsom salt first*** and slowly increase over several weeks.

3. 5-Hydroxytryptophan or 5HTP

Your body makes 5HTP from tryptophan, which is an amino acid. The 5HTP is then used to make serotonin.

Our body naturally makes melatonin from serotonin at night, which makes us get sleepy. Melatonin is a brain chemical signal that regulates our circadian rhythm.

5-HTP supplements are often used to help reduce stress, improve mood, and sleep quality.

Taking a 5HTP supplement at night will help boost melatonin levels at night to treat sleep disorders like insomnia.

5-HTP is generally preferred over L-tryptophan because it crosses the blood-brain barrier at a higher rate, and is converted into serotonin more efficiently than L-tryptophan.

Young children may take 50mg of 5-HTP before bed. And older children may take up to 100 mg.

4. Melatonin

If 5HTP didn't work for you for sleep, you could try melatonin supplements at bedtime. Melatonin is a natural sleeping aid that our body makes at night. Children with ADHD tend to have lower melatonin as well.

Our body makes melatonin from 5HTP naturally in the pineal gland located in the brain base. It controls the circadian rhythm – our body's biological clock that controls when you wake up, and when you should sleep.

Our body makes more melatonin as the day gets darker to calm and induce sleepiness. As the day starts in the morning, cortisol, the wake-up hormone, takes over.

Melatonin makes you fall asleep and stay asleep at night so that you wake up in the morning refreshed and alert.

When my daughter was ten years old, she seemed to be tired all the time. She was always falling asleep in short car rides (5-10 minutes). She can sleep for over 10 hours if she is given the time and allow her to do so. I suspected that she must not be sleeping well. She always wakes up still tired even after 10-12 hours of sleep.

One night I decided to let her try melatonin. She fell asleep a lot quicker than usual, without the usual tossing and turning and wanting to play more. We tried this for about a week. Some days, she can wake up on her own in the morning, which is unusual.

She was also able to verbalize that with the melatonin, she can "organize" her thoughts better during the day. My reaction was "wow," that was quite some interpretation and observation.

You may start with 5mg every night before bed. It does not make you feel drowsy or groggy at like many prescription sleeping pills.

EAT TO FOCUS QUICK START GUIDE

1. Get The Whole Family Involved

Announce to your family your intention for lifestyle changes and ask for their support. Then explain to your child with ADHD how this will benefit them now and in the future. Expect moaning, crying, and complaints. But you know this is best for your family.

Ask to try for at least one month. Sit down as a family to plan out next week's meals - breakfast, lunch and dinner, and snacks. Look up "plant-based recipes," Each family member picks an item or two for the week.

This is the rule to follow. Each family member picks a meal item. This member will prepare the shopping list and supervise the preparation of this meal. The rest of the family will support this member by enjoying the finished product (whether good or bad) with gratitude and appreciation for this member's effort.

This is how you create a pleasant mealtime together. Focus on the enjoyment of preparing a meal as a family, instead of that "I don't like that."

Do you rather eat a piece of bread and butter in a beautiful tranquil, scenic site? Or steak and lobster in a war zone?

2. Give Them a Sense of Control

In my years of working as a pediatric nutritionist, I realized that kids are picky with food is not so much about taste, but control. And poor parents try all kinds of tricks, search high and low for the perfect recipes to please their picky eater's palate.

Instead, all you have to do is give your child a sense of control within your boundaries.

Ask them what they want for dinner. Give them 2-3 choices to choose from. You remain in control of the choices, but your child feels a sense of control because he or she gets to pick.

Parents' job is to provide an environment for your child that is nurturing and nourishing. Children's job is to make good choices from their environment. When you surround your child with only good choices, he or she will only make good choices.

3. Stop Saying, "NO!"

When your child asks for something you don't want them to have, don't say "no." How many times your "no" has turned into a temper tantrum? And you ended up giving in because you can't stand your child screaming and crying.

Offer them an alternative that is approved by you, such as "how about we make some ants on logs for snack together" instead of chocolate chip cookies he or she asks for.

Speaking of which, if you don't want your child to have chocolate chip cookies, don't have them in the house.

Eliminate all the food you don't want your child to have from the house. Sit down with your child to come up with a list of new healthy snack ideas.

Use Pinterest to search for new recipes. Kids love pictures. Without the junk food in the house, you'll not have to say "no" again.

One parent told me she simple told her toddler that "we're not allowing to buy cookies." That's it. And her daughter stopped asking for cookies.

Are you smarter than a toddler?

4. Be the Change You Wish to See in Your Child

Children learn many of their habits and beliefs from the people closest to them, their friends, parents and families.

Many families fail to help their children eat better and achieve better weight because the parents are not willing to change.

When these families come to see me for their children's weight problems, they see it as their children's problem, not theirs.
But where does your child learn their eating habits, and when your child snack on junk food all day long, does your child go grocery shopping and buy all that junk food themselves?

And why are your children snacking on junk food all day long, where is the adult supervision?

Changes start with you, the parent.

5. Take Responsibility for Your Actions

If you want your child to eat fruits and vegetables and try new things, you have to be the change you wish to see in your child.

Parents' job is to provide a nurturing environment, which includes the food environment. Parents should provide the right kind of food that supports healthy growth and development. It is the child's job to pick and choose when he or she wants to eat.

I recently saw a boy for obesity. Mom keeps repeating that he is not picky. He would eat fruits, vegetables, and other healthy food. But he would refuse mom's homemade healthy lasagne. Why? Because he knows there's mac n cheese available in the house, and he knows his parents would let him have it.

I told the mom, he is not picky. He chose not to eat the dinner food because he knew there's something else he likes better available. If the mac n cheese weren't available in the house, he would have eaten the homemade lasagne just fine. And if his parents were more firm, they'd not have allowed him to eat the mac n cheese instead.

This is a problem of a lack of parental boundaries.

Who's running this household?

6. Be Flexible and Accept Failures

"I have not failed. I've just found 10,000 ways that won't work." Thomas A. Edison

Failure is part of the process. It's okay to fail. So instead of giving yourself permission to give up, permit yourself to fail. To succeed in any life situation, you have to be okay with failure.

Fall nine times, and get up the 10th time!

Expect that not every meal will be perfect. Like your previous diet, you don't always cook your steak perfect and don't always have your lasagne come out perfect. But you don't quit making steak or lasagne just because they didn't come out right the first time, right?

Accept that failure and mishap in the kitchen are part of life. I almost always burn my toast in the toaster. Instead of giving up eating toast, I now stand next to the toaster to watch my toast turn to the perfect shade I wanted and take it out promptly before it burns.

Think about the lessons learned and how you can become better because at it. It is these experiences that make you a better person.

Life is short, or long, and being grateful will help you appreciate all you have instead of focusing on what you don't have.

7. Be adventurous

Make every day a mini adventure of new favors and new texture. Try new ethnic foods and experiment with different spices and herbs.

Many ethnic foods are traditionally plant-based. In our household, we eat a variety of American, Japanese and Middle Eastern foods, and sometimes just baked fish with a mix-and-match of random herbs and spices, with a side of steamed vegetables seasoned with grass-fed butter salt and pepper, and potatoes for starches.

Dinner becomes a little surprise when your mix-and-match random herbs and spice that turns out very delicious. Just be creative and enjoy the journey.

Eating real food will take more effort. Don't think it won't. However, when you learn how to meal plan, use a cooking day, or find restaurants where you can get real food, it will be easy, worth it, and you won't look back.

8. Avoid Processed Food.

Processed food not only has no nutritional value but also contains artificial food additives and preservatives that interfere with hormonal and brain signaling.

Processed food also causes systemic inflammatory responses that result in behavioral changes, tantrums, anger outbursts, and meltdowns.

These foods include any processed food that comes out from a can, box, or package, fast food, fruit juice, sugar-sweetened beverages, and frozen meals.

9. Avoid Processed Fast Carbs

Carbohydrates are found in the following foods:
- All vegetables
- All fruits (except avocado) and juices
- Rice, grains, cereals, granola and pasta
- Bread, tortillas, crackers, bagels, and rolls
- Milk and yogurt
- Dried beans, split peas, and lentils
- Potatoes, corn, yams, peas, and winter squash
- Sweets and desserts, such as sugar, honey, syrups, pastries, cookies, soda, juices, and candy

Not all carbs are created equal. There are good carbs and bad carbs. And there are also fast carbs and slow carbs.

Fast carbs are foods that spike blood sugar. The ADHD brain has difficulty processing carbs and sugar. Therefore, eating food that causes a surge of sugar into the body will affect brain functions.

Avoid food on this list below:
- ***Cakes, cookies, candies, pastries, rice***, pasta, noodle, bread, chips, crackers, granola, cere-

al, desserts, *and fruit snacks have excessive sugar levels.*
- *All regular sodas, energy drinks, juice, and sugar-sweetened beverages, such as sweet tea, sweetened iced tea, flavored coffee, etc.*
- *Table sugar, honey, or any syrup. Natural sugars are still sugar.*
- *Fruit juices, soda, sugar, syrups, and candy can raise blood sugar quickly in less than 15 minutes. Therefore, it should be avoided at all costs.*

10. Eat Slow Carbs

Slow carbs even mood and energy, meaning fewer anger outbursts and emotional meltdowns, and more extended sustainable focus and concentration.

These include all your wholesome fruits and vegetables with natural carbs and sugar, and dietary fiber. Even starchy vegetables, such as potatoes, sweet potatoes, pumpkins, and squashes, are okay to eat.

The fiber content in these food helps to slow down the speed of sugar entering the bloodstream, which provides a longer sustainable source of energy without blood sugar spikes or crashes.

However, do limit fruits to no more than *three servings per day, only eat one serving at a time and always eat fruits with a protein or fats.*

Replace regular grain noodles with spaghetti squash, veggie noodles (zoodles) or Shirataki yam noodles (sold in Asian grocery stores and some natural food stores).

Replace rice with sweet potatoes, zucchini, pumpkin, yellow squash, butternut squash.

Also try *cauliflower mash, cauliflower pizza crust*.

With some creativity, you'll significantly reduce your grains intake while satisfying your cravings for pizza, cookies, pancakes, and waffles.

11. Mask Your Carbs

Always eat any food or beverage that can be converted to sugar with protein and fats. The higher protein and fat will "mask" the carbs at each meal and snacks and help prevent blood sugar spikes, which often leads to crashes. This way the body does not get overwhelmed with the massive load of carb or sugar coming in.

The protein and fats also help keep you feel fuller longer and avoid sugar cravings between meals.

People are often misguided by food manufacturers to think that carb is the only source of energy or fuel. The truth is your body can use fat and protein for energy between meals as well.

Examples are apple slices with almond butter, chicken or turkey breast with grapes, full-fat coconut yogurt with fresh berries, beef jerky with fruits, and tuna with cucumber/celery, etc.

By adding protein and fats to the mix, you're slowing down the carbs even more.

12. Eat Ingredients for Snacks

Raw fruits and veggies with natural organic beef jerky, full-fat coconut yogurt and boiled eggs or nuts (if tolerated after re-introduction) are excellent snack choices.

**See Bonus Chapter on *Fun and Delicious ADHD-Friendly and Kids-Friendly Snack Ideas*

13. Buy in Bulk

When there is a good deal or when something is especially delicious, stock up. Even fresh organic fruits and vegetables. Eat whatever you can fresh before they go bad, and freeze the rest for later use. Most fruits and vegetables keep well in the freezer, and you will always have them on hand.

Don't be ashamed to use frozen fruits and vegetables. They're just as nutritious. **Use frozen peas or frozen mixed veggies instead** when you don't have time to slice fresh veggies for a salad or to pack for lunch. They will be defrosted by lunch. Just top with your favorite dressing.

14. Dust off Your Slow-cooker or Pressure Cooker

They both do the same thing - make you dinner. One does it quickly, and one does it slowly. It's your choice. Either way, you'll enjoy a great meal.

Just throw in a bunch of your favorite veggies, herbs, tomatoes, and unprocessed meat, turn the dial on. Your dinner will be ready in no time with a pressure cooker, or after your nap if you're using a slow cooker.

15. Follow a meal plan

How many times have you try to make dietary changes and ended up giving up because you run out of recipes ideas or simple not knowing what to eat for breakfast, lunch and dinner.

Making dietary and lifestyle changes can be overwhelming when you have to search and experiment with new recipes.

However, having a meal plan to follow solves this dilemma while saving you tones of time, money and stress.

Having your meals planned out in advance is an excellent way to ensure you'll be fed well because you no longer say "I have no idea what to make for dinner" or "I forgot to pick up grocery" or "no time to make dinner," and end up eating cup noodle or ordering pizza again for dinner.

My patients use an easy-to-use meal planning app from RealPlans.com. You can customize the meal plan to your preference.

With the RealPlan apps, you create a meal plan you love and enjoy while following a healthy diet of real foods.

Download the 28-day meal plan here to try it out —> https://realplans.com/aip-meal-plans/free/?AFFID=432954

16. Create a grocery list.

Start your grocery store trip in the produce aisle. *Only shop on the outside perimeter of the store.* This is where this good stuff is. This helps eliminate most processed foods that you don't need.

Your cart should be filled with real fresh foods, not packaged foods.

If you use a meal planning app, such as RealPlan, the grocery list is automatically created based on the meals for the week and is ready on your phone app when you're in the grocery store.

You can check off the items you already have so you don't get too much.

17. Designate one day of the week to prepare "food for the week."

Who wants to cook dinner every single night?

Turn on some good music and invest an hour or two to prepare the meals and snacks for the coming week. Store individual meal portions in the freezer. It's kind of like making your own frozen meals.

Take one portion out in the morning and place in the refrigerator. When you come home for dinner, just heat it, and dinner is ready.

If you made multiple entrees, then you'll have different choices to choose from.

Don't forget to make enough for lunch too.

18. Avoid Sugar-free Food and Beverages

"Sugar-free" food only means no sugar added, but the item may still contain natural sugars from other ingredients, such as milk sugar and flour.

Products containing sugar-alcohols are often labeled "sugar-free," but they may still have significant amounts of total carbohydrate. *Look at the food label to see the grams of total carbohydrate =contained*.

Too much sugar alcohols may cause diarrhea or gas, and bloating. The following are examples of sugar-alcohols: hydrogenated starch hydrolysate (mixtures of sugar alcohols such as sorbitol, maltitol, and other sugar alcohols), isomalt, mannitol, sorbitol, xylitol.

19. Drink Water as Main Source of Hydration

Your body is made up of 70% water. So if you think eating the right food is important, then drinking pure water is even more so.

Water helps to flush out toxins from your liver and kidney. Just like the toilet tank needs to have water to flush your toilet, your body needs water to flush out toxins. That's a natural, everyday process, essential for life.

In that case, would you flush your toilet with sewer?

Choose pure water, unflavored bubbly water, and unsweetened brewed tea. You may flavor your water naturally with slices of citrus, berries, pineapple, cucumber, mint leaves, basil leaves, etc.

Avoid distilled water because distilled water pulls electrolytes or minerals from the body. Remember kids with ADHD frequently have low minerals so you want to avoid distilled water that pulls minerals from the body.

20. Keep a Food & Symptoms Journal

Keeping a food and symptoms journal helps to identify trouble food and track progress so you know what's working and what's not.

Start the first day eating like normal without making any changes or activities. Record everything eaten and the time eaten. Also record any physical symptoms, such as complain of stomach pain, frequently bowel movement including color consistency; and behaviors such as anger, tantrums, grumpiness, sleepiness, etc.

People often think "passing out" after eating is normal. The truth is that's not normal. Food is suppose to provide energy. If you or your child "pass out" after eating means the body has to use an extraordinary amount to break down the last meal, which means either the meal is too much or contains food that the body cannot handle and it's using all its resources to try to get rid of it.

21. Have fun.

This is my most favorite steps. Make eating healthy and clean fun is the best and most effective way to get your child, even picky eater, eats just about anything happily with a big smile.

Remember when your child used to be a baby crawling on the floor, and he or she would pick up random trash and put into their mouths?

I'm sure those trash does not taste even half as good as your food, but they are willing put it in their mouth because there's no pressure to eat. It's just fun exploration.

Parents often wants to do everything for their kids - prepare and cook all the meals, plate them for them, etc.

Let your child help with meal planning, grocery shopping and meal preparation. Let them choose the between a few pre-determined entree and have them help out in the kitchen. For older kids, they can help prepare the grocery list, clean and prepare ingredients and set up the table.

Younger children can help wash and clean ingredients, take things out from refrigerator, hand you utensils, toss in ingredients and even press a few buttons on appliances.

Make them part of the process while teaching them responsibility and helping around the house.

Kids are more likely to consume and try things they help prepare.
Well, that's is it.

Parenthood is the most beautiful thing. You bring a new human being into this world, and the most rewarding thing you can do for this little person is to nourish his/her body, mind, and soul.

Treat your child like how you'd like to be treated, and everything will be fine.

Thank you for going on this wonderful journey with me.

I hope you have enjoyed this book…

If you find this book life-changing, or at least enjoyable, please share it with your family, friends and associates and other parents of kids with ADHD to help them out.

If you would like further guidance or consultation with myself, please schedule a free consultation at https://anna-tai.lpages.co/contact/

Don't forget to leave a positive review on amazon.com or [Facebook page](#) to help out other parents like you.

Sharing is caring…

God bless!

ADDITIONAL RESOURCES

Don't forget to follow us on:

Facebook @*NaturalAlternativeADHDTreatment*

and

Pinterest @NaturalADHDStrategies *for more ideas and recipes.*

And join our FREE Facebook Private Support Group and hang out with other people who are working and playing with this material.

https://www.facebook.com/groups/628237007698227/

Visit *Natural-Alternative-ADHD-Treatment.com for new blog posts.*

For products and services mentioned in this book, check out the Resources page at:

https://natural-alternative-adhd-treatment.com/resources/

I'll be updating the resources there on an ongoing basis. So check back often and be sure to subscribe for updates.

To work with me, visit our Services page at:

https://natural-alternative-adhd-treatment.com/services/

Appendix

FOOD INTAKE & SYMPTOM TRACKER

Time	Food Eaten (include ingredients)	Behaviors	Digestive Symptoms

FOOD INTAKE & SYMPTOM TRACKER

Time	Food Eaten (include ingredients)	Behaviors	Digestive Symptoms

FOOD INTAKE & SYMPTOM TRACKER

Time	Food Eaten (include ingredients)	Behaviors	Digestive Symptoms

FOOD INTAKE & SYMPTOM TRACKER

Time	Food Eaten (include ingredients)	Behaviors	Digestive Symptoms

FOOD INTAKE & SYMPTOM TRACKER

Time	Food Eaten (include ingredients)	Behaviors	Digestive Symptoms

FOOD INTAKE & SYMPTOM TRACKER

Time	Food Eaten (include ingredients)	Behaviors	Digestive Symptoms

FOOD INTAKE & SYMPTOM TRACKER

Time	Food Eaten (include ingredients)	Behaviors	Digestive Symptoms

Brain Kryptonite Food to Avoid During Clean Start

This list contains food and ingredients that will directly or indirectly interfere with your child's brain chemical pathways.

Here's the *beginner's list of foods to avoid…*

- **Processed Meats** such as bacon, ham, pastrami, salami, pepperoni, chorizo, hot dogs, hot dogs, ham, bacon and turkey bacon, corned beef, pepperoni, salami, smoked turkey, bologna and other luncheon and deli meats, corned beef, biltong, canned meat, spam, chicken nuggets, etc.

- **Eggs**: whole eggs, egg yolks, egg whites, cooked eggs, cholesterol-free eggs, custard, cakes, cookies, eggnog, meringue, mayonnaise, Caesar salad dressing, Hollandaise sauce, nougat, pasta noodle, lysozyme, ovalbumin, surimi, albumin, egg substitutes, ice cream, lecithin, marzipan, marshmallows, nougat.

- **Cow's milk:** butter, butter fat, cheese, cottage cheese, sour cream, creams, ice cream, sherbet, pudding, custard, frozen desserts, goat milk, margarine, mayonnaise, buttermilk, whey or whey products, cow's milk yogurt, evaporated milk, powdered milk, chocolate, nougat, donut, mashed potatoes, processed meats, cold cuts, deli meat, salad dressing, artificial butter or cheese flavor, casein or caseinates, curd, ghee, hydrolysates, lactalbumin, lactalbumin phosphate, lactose, lactoglobulin, lactoferrin, lactulose, rennet.

- **Grains**: amaranth, barley, buckwheat, bulgur, corn, einkorn, farro, freaked, Kamut, millet, oats, quinoa, rice, rye, sorghum, spelt, teff, wheat, and wild rice.

- **Nuts**: all nuts and nut butters made from almonds, Brazil nuts, cashews, hazelnuts, pecans, pistachios, and walnuts.

- **Legumes**: garbanzo beans, black beans, kidney beans, mung beans, lima beans, chickpea, black-eyed peas, lentils, snow peas, sugar snap peas, peanuts, soybeans, tofu, soymilk, white beans, pinto beans, fava beans.

- **Processed refined carbs**: rice, pasta, noodle, cookies, crackers, chips, candies, chocolate candies, cereal, granola, fruit snacks, desserts, fruit juices, soda or pop, table sugar, syrup, high fructose corn syrup, etc

- **Processed refined sugars, sweets & desserts:** sugar is almost all man-made and should be avoided at all costs. The rule of thumb here is, if it has sugar listed as an ingredient, it is "added sugar" and should be avoided.

- **Artificial Sweeteners**: table sugar, agave, candy, chocolate, corn syrup, high fructose corn syrup, sucrose, and non-nutritive sweeteners: acesulfame potassium, aspartame, neotame, saccharin, sucralose.

- **Sugar alcohol:** mannitol, sorbitol, xylitol, lactitol, isomalt, maltitol and hydrogenated starch hydrolysates (HSH)

Other food items to avoid: Gluten-containing compounds: barbecue sauce, binders, bouillon, cold cuts, condiments, emulsifiers, fillers, chewing gum, hydrolyzed plant and vegetable protein, textured vegetable protein, ketchup, malt and malt flavoring, malt vinegar, matzo, meat glue, modified food starch, monosodium glutamate, nondairy creamer, processed salad dressings, seitan, some spice mixtures, stabilizers, soy sauce, teriyaki sauce.

Rocket Fuel for the ADHD Brain

ORGANIC MEATS & ORGANS
Almost all-natural meats are allowed. You'll want to stay away from highly processed meats. Choose organic meats as much as possible to avoid pesticides, antibiotics, and growth hormones.
- Poultry
- Turkey
- Chicken
- Pork
- Beef
- Lamb
- Fish
- Shrimp
- Lobster
- Clams
- Salmon
- Venison
- Buffalo
- Goat
- Scallops
- Oysters
- Mussels
- Crab
- Abalone
- Sardines
- Salmon
- Tilapia
- Red snapper
- Mahi mahi
- Mackerel

- Halibut
- Haddock
- Anchovies
- Bass
- Eel
- Cod
- Bone broth, liver, hearts, sweetbread (the organ), bone marrow

SEEDS
- Macadamia nuts
- Pine nuts
- Pumpkin seeds
- Sunflower seeds

SLOW CARB VEGETABLES

Almost all vegetables are allowed, except corn, and canned vegetables. Choose organic vegetables as much as possible to avoid exposure to pesticides and other environmental toxins.

- Acorn Squash
- Asparagus
- Avocado
- Artichoke hearts
- Arugula
- Beets
- Beet greens
- Bell peppers
- Bok choy
- Broccoli

- Brussels sprouts
- Butternut Squash
- Cabbage
- Carrots
- Cauliflower
- Celery
- Chives
- Cucumbers
- Eggplant
- Green Onions
- Garlic
- Kale
- Kohlrabi
- Leeks
- Lettuce
- Mustard greens
- Olives
- Onions
- Parsley
- Peppers
- Plantain
- Potatoes
- Pumpkin
- Radishes
- Rhubarb
- Sea vegetables
- Shallots
- Spinach
- Squash
- Sweet Potato and yams (not real potatoes)
- Tigernut
- Tomatoes

- Water chestnuts
- Watercress
- Zucchini

SLOW CARB FRUITS

Fruits contain fructose (sugar from fruits), which is not the same as the processed sugar, "high fructose corn syrup." Fruits are great for your body because they are loaded with vitamins, minerals, and antioxidants, but they're also easy to overdo.

Avoid eating fruits in huge quantities as fruits are high in fructose. Try to limit to 3 servings of fruit a day, except lemon, limes, and avocado. Always eat fruits with protein and fats.

- Apples
- Apricot
- Avocado
- Banana
- Blackberries
- Blueberries
- Boysenberries
- Cherries
- Coconut
- Cranberry
- Grapefruit
- Jackfruit
- Kiwi
- Kumquat
- Lemon

- Lime
- Mandarin orange
- Nectarine
- Papaya
- Passionfruit
- Peaches
- Pears
- Pineapple
- Plum
- Orange
- Raspberry
- Rhubarb
- Strawberry
- Tangelo
- Tomatillo

FERMENTED FOODS

Fermented food and beverages are great for gut health. Try to include at least one of the following item a day.

- coconut milk kefir (fermented coconut milk)
- coconut yogurt (guar gum-free)
- ginger beer or ginger ale
- kimchi (Korean fermented Chinese cabbage)
- kombucha (fermented tea)
- sauerkraut (German fermented cabbage)
- water kefir (fermented water)

ORGANIC UNPROCESSED FATS AND OILS

I can't emphasize enough the importance of natural healthy fats in our diets. Children, especially children with ADHD, need even more fats because of brain defects in processing sugar as energy.

Contrary to popular belief, fat and oils do not make us fat. The human body relies on fats between meals to stabilize blood sugar and sustain energy, which stabilizes mood.

- Avocado Oil
- Avocado
- Coconut oil
- Extra virgin olive oil
- Lard
- Confit
- Tallow
- Palm oil (not palm kernel oil)
- Truffle oil

COCONUT
- coconut aminos
- coconut milk (guar gum-free)
- coconut water
- coconut water vinegar
- coconut cream (not concentrate)
- coconut oil

NATURAL SWEETENERS (use in moderation only)
- Stevia
- Monk Fruit

- Maple syrup
- Raw honey
- Blackstrap molasses
- Coconut sugar
- Date sugar

UNREFINED SEA SALT
- Celtic salt
- Himalayan Pink Salt
- Hawaiian Sea Salt

Fun & Delicious ADHD-Friendly & Kid Friendly Snacks

Every kid loves snacks. It's always the most exciting events of the day, I always encourage parents to *turn snack time into a fun activity to introduce new foods.*

Switching to the clean lifestyle can be challenging for kids. To help ease the transition, we start with snack, the most favorite activity of all kids.

The idea is really simple.

When my daughter was 4 years old, we decided to travel back home to Macau to visit my family. On the way back to Honolulu, HI, we're waiting at the Hong Kong International Airport terminal. *We're exhausting from traveling.*

My husband and I just like any parents would, just sat and chill within sight distance of our daughter. *Being her usual active self, she was running around climbing on seats and looking for trouble*. As long as she didn't walk over anyone I'm watching.

Next moment was the scariest moment of any moms. She found the trash can. Not just any trash can. It's the ones with the ashtray on top. I saw her *reached up her little hands and grab something from the ashtray and put in her mouth.*

I jumped up from my seat and dash to her as fast as I could possibly can. There's no way I could have reach her quick enough to stop her. By the time I get to her, she has already swallow that piece of trash.

I have no idea what she ate.

What I know was the bacteria she ingested. For sure, she got sick immediately after coming home. I told the doctor what happened, and he did a stool test. It's campylobacter.

In case, you didn't get my point.

Your child will eat anything on their own terms when it's fun and no pressure, even if it's garbage. And I know my cooking tastes better than garbage.

But she rather eats garbage than my food, that hurts.

I know how easy it is to grab a couple packages of animal crackers, goldfish crackers, pretzels and fruit snacks in case your kids got hungry.

The whole idea of Eat to Focus is to *switch from eating fake food that not only have NO nutritional value to eat whole real food*.

Now it's time for you to make the change.

So you're ready to get your child to eat some healthy and fun snacks?

Here are 24 ADHD-friendly and kid-friendly snacks ideas for your kiddo and you to enjoy.

Remember some of these ingredients are allowed if tolerated after re-introduction.

Fruits and nuts
- Apple slices and nut butter (not peanut)
- Blueberries and almonds
- Banana slices and nut butter (not peanut)
- Strawberries and macadamia nuts
- Sliced banana with nut butter and unsweetened coconut flakes
- Homemade trail mix (combine your favorite nuts, seeds, and dried fruit)

Veggies & Dips
- Celery and nut butter (not peanut)
- Carrots and nut butter (not peanut)
- Bell pepper and guacamole dip
- Carrots and guacamole dip
- Cucumber and guacamole dip

Lunch or Snacks
- Unprocessed turkey slices with sliced jicama
- Lettuce wraps with avocado and unprocessed turkey
- Deviled eggs (use avocado in place of mayonnaise)
- Cantaloupe slices wrapped in Prosciutto

- Chicken salad (cubed chicken with mashed avocado) in a lettuce wrap
- Sliced grapes and cubed chicken with mashed avocado

<u>Dessert Snacks</u>
- Coconut milk yogurt with frozen berries sweetened with stevia or monk fruit
- Peaches with coconut cream (whip coconut milk in the same way you'd whip heavy cream to make non-dairy coconut milk cream)
- Power balls (nut butter, dried fruit, and coconut flakes, mixed together and formed into balls)
- Fat bombs (coconut oil, cacao powder, almond butter, stevia or monk fruit; mix well, pour in ice cube, and freeze)
- Strawberries and dark chocolate
- Smoothie (frozen fruit, coconut milk, greens)
- Chia seed pudding (chia seed in nut milk sweetened with stevia or monk fruit)

Now look at this list, and see how many of these ADHD approved snacks you can make.

I can hear some of you say, "my child would not eat that."

Yes. Just by you saying that statement, you already made the decision for your child.

I've seen many picky eaters in my practice. I've seen it all, if you really think your child's picky eater is so bad, he or she would have seen a specialist like myself.

Many times, parents created the picky eating. If you offer your child broccoli once, and he or she refuses, and you concluded, "he does not like broccoli" and never offer broccoli again, your child will never learn to eat and like broccoli.

Do you rather be spending time with your child making these fun and yummy snacks together? Or do you rather take time off from work for the hundredth time to pick up your child from school for therapy or worse because your child's school call to tell you that your child bit another kid and they're calling the police on your 6-year-old?

The choice is yours.

BONUS CHAPTERS

"If you want more, you have to require more from your-self..."
Phil McGraw

How to Get Your Picky Eater to Eat Anything?

Seriously, anything.

When it comes to picky eaters, most parents have been told, "When they're hungry, they'll eat". But there are a few really, really, really stubborn children that hunger does not bother them, and some just thinks that "your food" is so disgusting that they rather starve themselves than to eat your food.

My daughter was a picky eater since the beginning. She would refuse the bottle, no matter what's in it, formula and even breastmilk. She would refuse food as well. She would starve herself during the day when I'm at work and wait until I come home to nurse her.

And when she did eat, she did not want to be fed, she wanted to do it herself. If you touched her spoon, she'd throw a fit and meal time was over.

Then when she's older, she would eat the same food every meal every day, and she'd taste any little changes you made to her food. She even tasted it when I used different oil in her noodle one time.

If you make her eat that one last piece of chicken, she would chew and chew forever with tears and then eventually she'll gag and throw up.

Feeding this child has always been a struggle. Every meal was a fight with yelling, shouting and crying.

The epiphany came one day when I threw in the towel. I was tired of fighting with her with no end in sight. I was tired of being the "bad mom" who forced her child to eat. So I let her eat whatever she wanted even if it's not the most nutritious food. I cringed, but whatever…she's eating.

From then on, she started eating not just the junk she likes, but also trying new foods on her own. She also learned to cook because she doesn't like my cooking 90% of the time.

There are only a handful of things I make that she'll eat, such as *homemade fresh tomato salsa, cold tofu salad, stir fry green beans with pine nuts, roasted broccolini, Chinese steamed fish,* etc.

Sounds familiar…

While working in Feeding Team *we keep seeing the same feeding mistakes parents make when trying to get their kids to eat more*, and here are the seven strategies that helped many of my patients to get their child to eat better.

These are the same techniques I get even the pickiest picky eaters like kids with autism or sensory processing disorder and even oral aversion to start eating real food.

One of my 3-year-old patient with autism started eating broccoli after our first visit. Mom was super excited as they've been in feeding therapy for years to get her to eat a bite of veggies.

As the caregiver, you play the biggest role in your child's eating behavior. What you say around food and do with food or mealtime has a huge impact on developing healthy eating habits.

Parents' responsibilities is to provide the right food and the right environment. It is your child's choices to choose to eat or not.

1. Understand that Eating is a Sensory Experience

Eating involves all 5 senses – how the food looks, how it smells, how it feels (when touching with your hands and how it feels inside your mouth), how it tastes, and how it sounds (when you bite or chew).

Think of the most disgusting things that someone makes you eat. Think poop. Do you want to look at it? Do you want to touch it? Do you want to smell it?

I know this is an extreme example, but that's how your child looks at some of the food.

That's right. If you can't even stand to the sight of the food or touching that food, it will not be consumed.

That's how your child think of the food you want him/her to try. I know you're not feeding your child poison, but that's what's going on in your child's head. He/She has already made a conscious decision about that food.

Your job as the parent is to change his/her thought about eating that particular food. Kids would do anything when it's fun, so your job is to make eating fun. Hopefully, he/she will start associating eating with fun memories and slowly forget about the old rules.

2. Adjust your Expectations.

Parent always say, "My child does not like broccoli. He tried it once and spit it out. So we stop offering it to him."

Parents have the misconception that if the child spits out the food or makes face that means they don't like it, and never serve that food again.

That's not true.

In infants, they spit out food because it is a new texture for them. They've been on a full liquid diet since birth, now you're giving them something thicker, of course, they need time to adjust.

Toddlers just don't have the manners to politely swallow the food even if they don't like the new food yet.

Remember when your children say "no" to everything? They don't know what they're talking about. They say "no" because they hear you say it all the time.

Kids do things to get attention and reaction from parents.

Spitting out food or grimacing just means your child did not like the food TODAY, not forever. Try it another time, prepare it differently and make it fun.

Parents always complain that their children would eat French fries, but not baked or mashed potatoes. Or would eat applesauce, but not apple slices.

To an adult, they are the same food – potatoes or apple. To a child, they are different food. Your young toddler does not know they come from same source because they are just cognitively not there yet to realize.

They look different, taste different, and they eat differently, and therefore, they are different.

As adult, when we try a new food, we mean taking a bite, chewing and swallowing the food even if it tastes bad. In some occasions, you may spit it out if it's really gross.

I just have some salad that did not taste all that great, but I chewed and tasted it, and finally swallowed it despite the bad taste.

In children, you have to change your expectation. The ***definition of trying may mean really just an attempt, such as touching the food, smelling it, kissing, licking***, or if your child takes a bite and spit it out. That's fine too.

Another mistake parents make is not offering new food because "they'll not eat anyway, why waste food."

The problem with this is you're teaching your child that he or she has his or her own food, and the rest of the family has their own food. You also take away opportunities for your child to make decision for themselves to try new food.

3. Make Eating a Fun Activity

I have many parents who told me how they ***absolutely would not eat certain vegetables*** because they were ***forced*** to eat them when they're little.

Please don't repeat history. Learn from your own experience.

Kids love candies and cakes not because they taste great, but because of the fun and excitement associated with these food.

Kids don't like vegetables because you never hear any parent says, "***If you stop crying, I'll give you a broccoli***." But what you hear a lot is, "***Eat your broccoli, otherwise, you're not leaving the table***."

Parents subconsciously introduce the idea that candies are fun and broccoli sucks. Of course, cakes are great because they're always decorated and surrounded by fun people and activities. And you never force them to eat cake. Who doesn't love cake?

You don't necessarily need to make meal time a party every day, but at least make it fun and hands on. Kids love touching with their hands and cause-and-effect activities.

Let them eat with their hands, smear food on dinner plates and on themselves, build towers, stick people, etc. Let them smell the food, kiss it, lick it. Take a tiny bite and spit out. That's all totally fine.

To most children, eating is just another activity, just like doodling, watching TV, reading, dancing, etc. For them, they are not getting as much enjoyment out of eating than, say, riding a bike. So eating is just not a priority. They want something more stimulating.

You can turn eating into an activity by getting your child involve in the shopping, meal planning and preparation. Give them age-appropriate task to help. Let them get hands-on with food, such as taking food out from refrigerator, mixing sauces or salads, cut fruits and veg with plastic knives, etc.

Turn these activities into fun family activities rather than treating these as chores. Give them a *sense of control* by letting them *pick from 2 predetermined healthy choices*.

True story...one day my daughter ask to bring a jar of Nutella to school. Curious, I asked why because she does not eat Nutella. She told me that she and her friends were each bringing something from home and mixing all the food together into a concoction and see how it would taste.

When I picked her up from school that day, she gave me a rundown of the all the food on their list. As she went through the list, I couldn't stop thinking why she would eat that "disgusting" mix than the food that I meticulously prepared for her. Then it dawned on me…because it is FUN.

My daughter is still very picky to this day, which forces her to be more involved in meal planning so she can make her own food when she doesn't like what I make. Again, I don't want to fight. I just want to enjoy a pleasant meal every day.

The saving grace is that my daughter loves fruits and vegetables. And she loves making food from scratch with fresh ingredients. So I'm happy as she's not loading on processed foods.

Give up your control, drop your expectations and let them be. Eating should be enjoyable for the whole family.

4. **Maintain a schedule meal and snack time**.

Many parents are so concern with their child "not eating" that they overcompensate by allowing their children free range to the pantry, and some even has a snack bowl on the coffee table accessible at all times by the child.

The children end up "grazing" all day long and, of course, they're not hungry at meal times for real food. Imagine yourself eating a few bites of food every hour. Would you still feel hungry at meals?

If you want your child to eat "real food", then you need to restrict snacks to only 1-2 times a day. And avoid snacking an hour before meals.

It's okay for your child to be hungry. Parents are so afraid that their children are hungry. Hunger is a normal human sensation just like thirst and other feelings. Children needs to learn the sense of hunger and how to appropriately response to it.

5. Always offer food first and give liquids toward end of meal or between meals.

Assuming you've put your children on a strict meal and snack schedule, your child should be hungry at meal times now. So take advantage of this hunger and offer real foods you want your child to try.

Hunger is your friend, offer new food when your child is hungry. You know you're less picky when you're hungry.

Don't let your child fill up with liquids, that'll ruin your plan. Liquids should be only for hydration and not a substitute for nutrition.

If your child depends heavily on liquid nutrition, you need a medical evaluation.

6. Limit mealtimes to no more than 30 minutes.

So many parents make the mistake of making their children sit at the table for an hour, sometimes up to 2 hours, in hope that their children will finish their food.

I'm guilty too…I used to make my daughter sat at the table until she finishes her last teeny bite of chicken with tears running down her cheeks.

Poor child…I didn't know better back then.

It's not pleasant for you or your child. It turns mealtime into a battle. And everyone is angry and frustrated.

Let me tell you this strategy does not work. The longer your children sit at the table the more everyone become frustrated and the less likely your child will eat. This only creates more tension at meal time.

Sing with me: "let it go…let it go…turn away and slap the (bathroom) door!"

7. Be a role model to your child.

Monkey see, monkey do.

Many parents tell me, "my child is only interested in the food on my plate, even if I gave him or her the same food I have on his or her plate."

Why?

Because they see how much you're enjoying your food, that's why they want your food. They're too young to realize that they have the same food on their plate.

If they see you grimace at eating healthy food, they'll learn to do the same.

It's totally okay for your child to reject new food initially. It's just that the sight, the taste, the texture are unfamiliar.

It's also okay if your child coughs, chokes or gags with new food. Stay calm as long as your child is not turning blue.

Your panicking can alarm your child and they may think something is wrong with them.

Every child is different. That's why you have children who are picky and some who are not. Some find more enjoyment in eating than others.

And here are six underlying causes of your child's extreme pickiness with food:

- Autism
- Sensory processing disorder
- Developmental disorders
- Food allergies
- Gastrointestinal disorders
- Constipation

When Should You Be Concern?

When I started working in the Feeding Clinic, I realized there are extreme picky eaters who would gag and vomit at the sight or smell of food, some would crawl under the table when they know it's meal time. And I've also seen kids whose diet involves only five food and they need a feeding tube to get the rest of the nutrition.

Here are other signs and symptoms that your child's extreme pickiness with food may need professional help:

- Your child coughs, chokes or gags when eating or drinking along with frequent respiratory illnesses.

- Your child's pickiness with food is affecting his/her growth.

- Your child have significant sensory issues, such as not transitioning to table food by 12 months of age.

- Your child's food choices continue to decrease with absolute no luck with new foods.

8 Brain Booster Supplements for ADHD

Supplements are one of my **favorite subjects** because I recommend supplements for my patients all the time.

If you go to any **regular dietitians or nutritionists, they'll freak out if you tell them that you take any kind of supplements**.

You'll be lectured on how "supplements are not regulated," "you're wasting money," because "none of the claims are proven or approved," and so on, and on...

On the other hand, I love them because, when you use the right supplements properly the way it's supposed to, *they're magical*.

Supplements are only useless if you don't need it or you're using the wrong ones.

Patients come to me with **all kinds of supplements they buy from GNC, Vitamin Shoppe, Whole Foods, and anywhere online.**

100% of the time, they don't know what's in it. All they know is that the sales clerk says, "it'll help with your [insert problem]."

Is the sales clerk a medical doctor or registered dietitian just working part-time at the store?

It bothers me that people would pay hundreds of dollars on useless supplements recommended by a sales clerk, who makes minimum wage to pay their rent than to spend that money on a specialist who knows their stuff and gets them to the results they want fast.

Then, they'll complain that the supplement does not work.

Duh?! What do you expect?

You'll save so much more money, frustration, and time with a specialist who can get you started on the right path right away.

Let's talk about some basics about supplements. They can be generally categorized into three types based on their purposes.

3 Purposes of Supplements:

1. To correct a nutrient deficiency
2. To boost a function
3. To correct a defective or weak biochemical pathway

1. *The first category is mostly your essential vitamins, minerals, and antioxidants that the human body needs.* These include vitamins A, B, C, D, E and K, magnesium, zinc, iron, alpha-lipoic acid, acetyl-L-carnitine, serotonin, melatonin, etc. These are what your body survives on.

2. *The second category includes nutrients like zinc to boost immunity, alpha-lipoic acid, coenzymeQ10, S-adenosyl-methionine, acetyl-L-carnitine to boost mitochondria (cell's powerhouse) function*, especially for someone on a ketogenic diet or high-fat diet.

3. *The third category is where all the other herbal supplements and anything else belongs.* These are your coffee, rhodiola, ginseng, ginkgo Biloba, ashwagandha, passionflower, etc. The body does not have an essential need for these herbal supplements, but they function as medicines to treat something.

Most children and adults can benefit from the vitamin-mineral-diet approach. But those with more significant ADHD may need more potent stuff like "herbs." These herbs are what I like to call "brain boosters."

Many medicines we use today come from plants. Pharmaceutical companies take the active compound out of the plant, tweak a couple of molecules, make them super powerful, put a patent on it, and bank on the exclusive right to sell the "new drug" for ten years.

Many parents might consider herbal supplements as safer alternatives. It is typically perceived as a gentle "natural medicine" with fewer side effects because it's natural, plant-based, and safe.

Being "natural" or "plant-based" does not make anything safer. As my pharmacist intern told me frequently, "Cyanide is natural. Will you take it?"

Many of these herbal supplements have actual medicinal properties, which means they can be as dangerous as any prescription drug.

Many pharmaceutical drugs we use today originally come from plants. For example, aspirin comes from the bark of the willow tree, or digitalis (heart medicine) comes from the dried leaves of the common foxglove (Digitalis purpurea).

That's why herbal supplements can be quite potent and dangerous if not used properly because they are real "medicine."

The natural herbs and spices we use for cooking are excellent because the amount we use in cooking is small.

But when these herbs and spices are ground up and stuffed into a pill form or tincture, these can become powerful medicine in a concentrated form.

Brain boosters are supplements that the body either makes and uses naturally or herbal supplements with medicinal properties.

Please be a smart cookie and check with your doctor before experimenting on these supplements, especially if you're already taking any prescription medications.

1. 5-Hydroxytryptophan or 5 HTP

5-HTP is used for treating many co-existing disorders of ADHD, such as sleep disorders, depression, anxiety, and obsessive-compulsive disorder (OCD), by increasing serotonin levels.

L-5-hydroxytryptophan (5-HTP) is the immediate precursor of serotonin (5 HT), a powerful neurotransmitter in your body. It is a chemical that exists naturally in your body. Your body makes 5-HTP naturally from tryptophan, an amino acid, from protein that you ingest. It is then converted into serotonin, which regulates memory, learning, mood sleep, appetite, temperature, sexual behavior, and pain sensation.

Low serotonin level is associated with poor memory, low mood, sugar/sweets cravings, sleep disorder, anxiety, and aggression.

Benefits of 5 HTP for ADHD

80-90% of your body's serotonin is made in your intestines. But serotonin cannot cross the blood-brain barrier. So all the serotonin that your brain needs has to be made within the brain. This is where 5-HTP comes into play.

5-HTP crosses the blood-brain barrier more readily than *tryptophan* and is then converted into *serotonin* in the brain faster than from tryptophan.

5 HTP works by increasing the production of serotonin in the brain and the central nervous system.

A study in 2011 looked at 85 children with ADHD between the ages of 4 and 18 who were treated with serotonin and dopamine amino acid precursor (5 HTP and L-tyrosine) protocol. In total, 67% of participants achieved significant improvement with only amino acid precursors of serotonin and dopamine at three weeks, and 77% improvement at eight weeks.

How to Supplement 5 HTP for ADHD?

5 HTP supplements should be taken with L-tyrosine, the precursor to dopamine.

When you take 5-HTP alone, you are depleting dopamine, norepinephrine, and epinephrine. The conversion to *serotonin from 5-HTP*, and *dopamine from L-DOPA* is catalyzed by the same enzyme, *L-aromatic amino acid decarboxylase (AAAD)*.

When you supplement 5 HTP without L-tyrosine, your body will use the AAAD enzyme to make serotonin and not enough to make dopamine and other catecholamines. Over time, you'll have a dopamine deficiency. Therefore, it's best to supplement 5 HTP with L-tyrosine to avoid dopamine deficiency.

The starting dose used in the study above is as follows:

For children 16 years and younger: 75mg 5 HTP and 750mg L-tyrosine twice a day

For children/adult 17 and older: 150mg 5 HTP and 1,500mg L-tyrosine twice a day.

Is 5 HTP Supplement Safe?

5-HTP is a natural substance in our bodies. Thus, it is generally safe to use for short-term up to 12 weeks.

5-HTP is a naturally occurring amino acid derived from seed pods of *Griffonia simplicifolia*, found in West and Central Africa. 5-HTP content in extracts of this plant varies from 2 – 20.83% (from seeds obtained in Ghana).

Make sure to look for pure 5-HTP or griffonia simplicifolia extract on the label.

Avoid taking 5-HTP if you're already taking antidepressants

Taking 5HTP with medications (such as an SSRI or MAOI) for depression might increase serotonin too much and cause serious side effects, including heart problems, shivering, and anxiety.

Some of these medications for depression include fluoxetine (Prozac), paroxetine (Paxil), sertraline (Zoloft), amitriptyline (Elavil), clomipramine (Anafranil), imipramine (Tofranil), and others.

If you're taking any of these medications and medications that help with moods, anxiety, and depression, check with your prescribing doctor to see if 5 HTP is beneficial for you.
Don't say I didn't warn you.

2. Alpha Lipoic Acid

Oxidative stress plays a crucial role in cognitive disorders and decline because nerve tissues are susceptible to free radical damage.

Accumulated oxidative damage to mitochondria in brain cells eventually leads to memory and brain function.

Oxidative stress happens when reactive oxygen species, or "free radicals," build up faster than antioxidants can work to quench them. It makes sense then that ingesting potent antioxidants that can readily cross the blood-brain barrier would aid in staving off or slowing some of the damage caused by oxidative stress.

The antioxidant alpha-lipoic acid has been found to improve memory and learning in mouse models. Mice are administered alpha-lipoic acid daily for 11 months of age and continuing until death.

A subset of 18-month-old mice given alpha-lipoic acid for two weeks and then tested in an object-place recognition paradigm had improved memory. The second subset of 18-month-old mice given alpha-lipoic acid for two weeks and tested in the Barnes maze had enhanced learning.

The mice that received alpha-lipoic acid had significantly higher glutathione and decreased glutathione peroxidase and malondialdehyde, indicating a reversal of oxidative stress. These results suggest that alpha-lipoic acid improves memory and reverses indices of oxidative stress in extremely old mice.

6 Benefits of Alpha Lipoic Acid for the ADHD Brain

The mechanisms by which ALA acts on the brain are many.

1. Alpha-lipoic acid boosts acetylcholine production, *a brain chemical related to memory creation and overall brain function.* Acetylcholine has an essential role in enhancing alertness when we wake up, sustaining attention, learning, and **memory**. ALA has also been shown to improve the function of brain chemicals, such as dopamine, serotonin, and norepinephrine.

2. Alpha-lipoic acid increases *glucose* uptake in brain cells, providing you with a boost of *mental energy*.

One of the ADHD brain defects is poor glucose metabolism. ALA increases glucose metabolism by enhancing glucose transport into cells and the activity of crucial enzymes for mitochondrial energy production.

Alpha-lipoic acid is used to break down carbohydrates and make energy for the other organs in the body.

3. Alpha-lipoic acid *regenerates other antioxidants. ALA is a potent antioxidant. It's* the ability to fight oxidative stress is many times more potent than other better-known antioxidants.

Because it regenerates other antioxidants depleted by the ongoing fight with free radicals, it allows you to use antioxidants *Vitamin C & E, glutathione* and *CoQ10* already in your body over and over again.

Low levels of glutathione are linked to many brain disorders, such as autism, ADHD, and schizophrenia.

4. *Alpha-lipoic acid improves cellular energy levels, which is the energy* behind every single action that happens in your body, including your brain. Cellular energy is required for muscle movement, producing new cells, wound healing, and *thinking*. The mitochondria are like the power station in your city. Every single cell in your body has many mitochondria to support its energy needs.

The mitochondria in each of your cells are the source of this energy. This ongoing energy production process is called the **Krebs Cycle**. Alpha-Lipoic Acid is an essential cofactor to two essential enzymatic reactions within the Krebs Cycle.

Mitochondrial function declines with age, meaning less energy is available for the brain cells. ALA can boost energy production in the mitochondria by increases glucose uptake in brain cells.

Alpha-lipoic acid improves energy production within the cell's mitochondria, aka the "powerhouse." This energy role may be one of the mechanisms involved in reducing dementia symptoms.

Further evidence that supplemental ALA helps mitochondrial function is demonstrated by patients with mitochondrial muscle disorders whose strength and energy levels improve with ALA supplementation.

5. ALA may help with heavy metal chelation. Exposure to high levels of environmental toxins, such as heavy metal, pesticides, polluted air, water, etc., increases oxidative damage to mitochondria in brain cells, eventually leading to nerve cells and cognitive dysfunction.

ALA chelates toxic heavy metals, while reducing inflammation, and cellular damage by heavy metals.

Studies show ALA helps clear neurotoxic heavy metals, including mercury. As you may know, mercury has been found in high levels in seafood and manmade products and can readily cross the blood-brain and placental barriers.

6. *ALA crosses the blood-brain barrier.*

Another *superpower of alpha-lipoic acid is that it can function in both fatty and water medium.*

Unlike other antioxidants like vitamin C, which works best in a water medium, and vitamin E works best in fatty medium ALA can work in both aqueous and fat mediums.

Because it can function in both the fatty and water medium, it can easily cross the blood-brain-barrier into the brain and eliminate cell-damaging toxins from the brain.

What are Sources Rich in Alpha Lipoic Acid?

It is always *a good idea to get your nutrients from fresh organic food sources* to get all the extra antioxidants that come with natural food.

Most people who do not have an aging brain function or Alzheimer's disease can probably get away with eating a healthy, clean diet with food that is naturally rich in alpha-lipoic acid.

However, for those with *poor memory or brain function, such as ADHD, brain fog, Alzheimer's, supplementation with alpha-lipoic acid is probably your best bet.*

How Much Alpha Lipoic Acid to Take a Day?

There is *no recommended dose of alpha-lipoic acid* from the US Food and Drug Administration because the body can make its own.

In a study in mice, it was found that the administration of *alpha-lipoic acid and acetyl-L-carnitine for two weeks was found to improve memory in mice.*

Another *study for Alzheimer's disease found that a daily intake of 600 mg alpha-lipoic acid slowed the disease's progression.*

These studies' results are likely related to the combined benefit of alpha-lipoic acid in stopping oxidative cellular damage and improving mitochondrial function.

Juvenon Pro Cognition from Douglas Laboratories provides a unique combination of alpha-lipoic acid, L-acetylcarnitine, and alpha-GPC that naturally improves focus and memory.

Is Alpha Lipoic Acid Safe?

No adverse effect has been reported on doses of up to 600mg per day for an adult.

3. Co-Enzyme Q10

Coenzyme Q10 or CoQ10 (for short) is an *antioxidant that our body makes naturally*. It is also found in many natural foods we eat every day.

What are the Symptoms of Coq10 Deficiency

Low levels of CoQ10 results in brain fog, slow mental processing, and cognitive decline.

CoQ10 deficiency is not that common because your body makes it.

If there's a deficiency, it's most likely due to stress, aging, drugs, and genetic mutation.

Your *body naturally makes less CoQ10 as you age*. And some people with *certain medical conditions may need more* than what the body can produce.

Stress in all forms, physical, mental, and emotional stress, illness increase the body's use of CoQ10.

Low blood CoQ10 levels have also been reported in people with heart diseases, gingivitis (inflammation of the gums), morbid obesity, muscular dystrophy, diabetes, AIDS, cancer, and some people on kidney dialysis.

What Does CoQ10 Do?

It is a *fat-soluble, vitamin-like substance that's found mostly in the mitochondria*, the body's power station. It is part of the electron transport chain and participates in aerobic cellular respiration to **make energy** in the form of ATP.

The **mitochondria are like the engine in the car. If it stops working, the car is dead.** CoQ10 is needed to convert carbohydrates and fats into energy in the inner mitochondrial membrane.

You'll *find mitochondria in every single cell of the body* because it is that important. And the organs that used the most energy, such as the brain, heart, liver, and kidneys, have the highest numbers of mitochondria AND concentration of CoQ10.

The mitochondria powers all the biochemical reactions in every cell of your body, and it cannot do its job correctly without CoQ10.

I talk to my teens every day about how important that they eat healthy food to feed their brain cells. We can eat all the fantastic, nutritious foods, but if our bodies can't turn these nutrients into energy, we're still doomed.

CoQ10 supports energy production in the mitochondria, which helps protect against brain degeneration. By supporting brain energy production, CoQ10 helps with neurotransmitters signaling and, thus, better memory, learning, and cognition.

Mitochondria are the powerhouses of the cell. They break down down nutrients from food and creates energy for the cell.

CoQ10 also protects against DNA, particularly mitochondrial DNA, damage from oxidative stress, which is common in most children with ADHD and Autism, and adults with Alzheimer's disease. This shows that CoQ10 can protect the degeneration of the brain cells due to aging.

Unlike other antioxidants, CoQ10 protects the body against the resultant oxidative stress from both the lipid peroxidation and protein oxidation. It also regenerates other antioxidants such as vitamin E.

What are Good Food Sources of CoQ10?

Rich sources of dietary coenzyme Q10 include mainly organ meats, meat, poultry, and fish. Remember always to get organic and grass-fed animal protein to minimize exposure to toxic pesticides, growth hormones, and unnecessary antibiotics.

Other good sources include soybean, corn, olive, and canola oils; nuts; and seeds. Fruit, vegetables, eggs, and dairy products are moderate sources of coenzyme Q10.

How to Get the Most out of Co10 to Boost Memory?

Studies show that taking CoQ10 supplements by mouth can increase mitochondrial concentrations in brain cells.

CoQ10 is fat-soluble, it's better absorbed when taken in an oil-based soft gel form than in a dry powder form, like powder tablets or capsules.

Dividing the total daily dosage up into two or more separate doses may also help with absorption.

There are mainly two forms of CoQ10 - ubiquinol, the active antioxidant form, and ubiquinone, the oxidized form. Our body can convert ubiquinone into ubiquinol (active form).

How Much CoQ10 to Take Daily?

The average dietary intake of coenzyme Q10 is about 3 to 6 mg/day, which is not enough to sustain adequate blood levels of CoQ10.

To get 30mg of CoQ10, you need to eat one pound of sardines, 2 pounds of beef, or two and a half-pound of peanuts.

People with specific health conditions may need higher levels.

Most of the *researches on heart diseases had used 90-150 mg* per day. The *typical recommended dosage for an adult is 30 mg to 300 mg daily*; higher daily intakes have been used in some studies.

How much CoQ10 does a child need?

There isn't a whole lot out there about how much coQ10 to supplement for a child. Ohio State University recommends *100mg/day for children with migraine headaches.*

4. Coffee

All ADHD medications such as *methylphenidate and amphetamines are stimulants, and so is caffeine, except caffeine does not need a prescription and readily available in beverages*.

How many people do you know drinks coffee every day? Like their lives depend on it?

Interestingly, *anecdotal evidence suggests that many people are already using caffeine to self-medicate themselves or their children.*

Coffee has long been known for its ability to increase alertness, reduce daytime tiredness, and improves mental focus and concentration.

Caffeine is the primary chemical compound that gives coffee its extraordinary power.

Caffeine has been studied for ages as a potential treatment for ADHD. But *its use as a "therapy" is not widespread because research studies show that it is less effective than the common stimulants used*.

However, one could have argued that the caffeine doses used in these studies were too low to have a consistent effect.

Of course, if caffeine is shown to be more effective or just as effective, pharmaceutical companies would lose customers to Starbucks.

Caffeine is probably one of the most consumed drug in the world — more than alcohol, and more than tobacco.

How Does Coffee Help ADHD?

Caffeine, or 1,3,7-trimethylxanthine, affects our brain chemistry by blocking the adenosine receptors in the brain. Adenosine is a central nervous system neuromodulator that binds to very specific receptors. *When adenosine binds to its receptors, neural activity slows down, making you feel tired and sleepy*.

Adenosine is not able to attach to its receptor by blocking the adenosine receptors, so you don't feel sleepy. By doing so, caffeine affects other neurotransmitters, such as dopamine, acetylcholine, serotonin, and norepinephrine.

The activation of numerous neural circuits by caffeine also causes the pituitary gland to secrete hormones that, in turn, cause the adrenal glands to produce more adrenalin. Adrenalin is the "fight or flight" hormone, which *increases your attention level and gives you an extra burst of energy*.

By affecting these other neurotransmitters, caffeine can deliver a major boost of energy to mental alertness even when we are well-rested.

By increasing dopamine transmission, *caffeine improves our mood and may protect brain cells from age- and disease-related degeneration*.

By increasing the activity of acetylcholine, *caffeine increases muscular activity and may also improve long-term memory.*

By raising and adjusting serotonin levels, *caffeine relieves depression, makes us more relaxed, alert, and energetic*, and it also *relieves migraine headaches* by causing constricting blood vessels in the brain.

In the ADHD brain, *stimulants, such as methylphenidate, amphetamines, and even caffeine, work by increasing dopamine levels and blocking the reuptake of norepinephrine.*

Many adults with ADHD symptoms are already using coffee daily to help them stay focus on tasks and get through the day.

Many people with ADHD function well enough with just caffeinated beverages to make it through life.

The cost of coffee is more affordable compare to expensive ADHD medication.

Not to mention all the *side effects of ADHD medications - anorexia, weight loss, loss of appetite, somnolence, sleep disturbance, tics, zombie-like...*

The use of caffeine does not have to be supervised by a health professional because it is not a dangerous controlled substance.

Did I mentioned that one possible side effect of ADHD medication is" *suicide ideation*"?

No, thank you...*I rather have a hyper and inattentive child than a suicidal one.*

And for some, they just *don't want to have to carry the burden of having a "mental" disorder*. Some occupations exclude candidates with any kind of mental disorder.

Caffeine certainly appears to be beneficial for some adults and children with ADHD. But just because it is easily accessible without a prescription, it is still a drug and does have side effects. Overconsumption and abusive use of anything (even if it's good) can be dangerous.

100 mg of caffeine is equivalent to the low therapeutic dose of 5 mg of Ritalin.

An 8-oz cup of brewed coffee has about 135 mg of caffeine, black tea 60 mg, green tea 30 to 40 mg, and most caffeinated sodas have 35 to 55 mg, and Red Bull energy drinks have up to 80 mg.

Does Coffee or Caffeine Make ADHD Worse?

Unlike conventional notions that caffeine makes you hyper, many people with ADHD find coffee to be calming and soothing. Some even become sleepy with coffee consumption.

Both caffeine and Ritalin are absorbed into the bloodstream within about 45 minutes and wear off after 3 or 4 hours.

Does Caffeine Cause Stunt growth?

The answer is no. John Hopkins just confirmed that. And I can also professionally testify from my experience. I've never seen a child with stunt growth from drinking coffee.

But ADHD medications…yes. I see that all the time.

How Much Caffeine Can a Child with ADHD Have?

I used to give my daughter about 4oz coffee in the morning before school and before tennis matches. And that's enough to help her focus.

You can experiment with the amount with your child, start with 1 ounce to see what happen.

If your child starts feeling jittery or shaky, then it's probably too much.

Use common sense to help your child.

There are other beverages that contain caffeine, but I find that caffeine from coffee works the best.

5. Ginseng

Ginseng is a very common herb used in Asian countries. You can find ginseng anywhere. When I was growing up Macau, my mom used to make ginseng chicken soup once in a while.

The chicken soup is always my favorite, but not when there's ginseng in it. The ginseng root adds a bitter flavor to the soup, but we're ordered to drink the whole bowl because "it's good for you."

So what's so good about ginseng?

Ginseng has many functions and benefits to our body and mind. First of all, it is an adaptogen, which means it helps the body adapt to stress by stimulating the immune system. There is also evidence that ginseng has anticarcinogenic and antioxidant properties.

Is Ginseng Good for ADHD?

Have you noticed that there's ginseng in many energy drinks on the market?

Ginseng doesn't improve physical performance, but it may boost your brainpower.

Ginseng, especially when used with Ginkgo biloba, is believed to improve focus and memory in children with ADHD.

Herbal extracts of ginseng are shown to target the brain's dopamine pathway and show a protective effect on these pathways from free radicals.

Ginsenoside, the active substance in ginseng, may help with some ADHD symptoms by boosting levels of dopamine and norepinephrine in the key brain regions that are affiliated with ADHD.

Interestingly, many stimulants used to treat ADHD also work by boosting levels of dopamine and norepinephrine.

Imbalances between dopamine and norepinephrine in children with ADHD are suspected as one of the causes of ADHD, resulting in disruptions of physiological processes such as attention span, complex cognitive processes, auditory processing delays, and motor behavioral dysfunctions.

Korean red ginseng can reduce the production of the adrenal corticosteroids, cortisol, and dehydroepiandrosterone (DHEA), and thus may be a viable treatment for ADHD.

A 2011 study showed that Korean red ginseng might be useful in improving inattentiveness in ADHD children. Eighteen children with ADHD aged between 6 and 14 were given Korean red ginseng (*Panax ginseng*) at 1,000 mg twice a day for eight weeks.

After eight weeks, significant differences were found in the omission errors of ADS, the Conners ADHD Rating Scale, and the Spielberger State Anxiety Scale.

In a 2014 study, children with ADHD between the ages of 6 and 15 were randomized into a Korean red ginseng group (n=33) or a control group (n=37). The KRG group received 1g KRG extract/pouch) twice a day, and the control group received one pouch of placebo twice a day.

At the eight week point, the primary outcomes were the *Diagnostic and Statistical Manual of Mental Disorders* (DSM-IV) criteria for inattention and hyperactivity scale scores, which were measured at baseline and eight weeks after starting treatment.

The KRG group had significantly decreased inattention/hyperactivity scores compared with the control group at week 8

A 2001 study looked at the combined effect of an herbal product containing American ginseng extract, Panax quinquefolium, (200 mg), and Ginkgo biloba extract (50 mg) for its ability to improve the symptoms of attention-deficit hyperactivity disorder (ADHD).

Thirty-six children with ADHD ranging in age from 3 to 17 years, took combines American ginseng and ginkgo Biloba capsules twice a day on an empty stomach for four weeks.

After two weeks of treatment, the proportion of the subjects exhibiting improvement ranged from 31% for the anxious-shy attribute to 67% for the psychosomatic attribute.

After four weeks of treatment, subjects showed improvements, such as a 44% improvement in the social problems and 74% for the Conners' ADHD index and the DSM-IV hyperactive-impulsive symptoms.

6. Gingko Biloba

How many times have you walked into a room and forgot what you're there for? Of misplaced your keys.

Or how many times you have to repeat yourself to your child because they keep forgetting what you just told them.

This herb may help.

You have probably heard about this super herb that helps with memory and focus. Research has shown that Ginkgo Biloba is a powerful herb for boosting memory and focus, which is just one of Gingko's many potential benefits.

Ginkgo has been used in Chinese medicine for thousands of years. It is traditionally used to treat respiratory issues such as asthma, wheezing, or coughing, incontinence, and digestive problems. It helps with depression and dementia, as well as inner ear problems such as tinnitus or vertigo.

Ginkgo biloba is also used extensively in Europe to treat dementia in Europe. And the American Geriatric Society has also stated that "Ginkgo biloba may help people who have Alzheimer's."

How Does Ginkgo Biloba Help with ADHD?

1. Ginkgo biloba protects the brain against degeneration as a powerful antioxidant. The active compounds of Ginkgo Biloba are a potent free radical scavenging agent and possess amazing antioxidant properties that protect the brain tissues from free radical damages.

2. Ginkgo biloba influences several brain chemicals. Ginkgo biloba is thought to boost the cholinergic processes in various cortical brain regions. Increases in cholinergic transmission are known to enhance working memory performance, while reductions in cholinergic transmission compromise performance on working memory tasks.

3. Ginkgo biloba boosts the nervous system by increasing blood flow and oxygen supply to the brain, which is frequently what the ADHD brain tends to lack. Ginkgo leaves contain substances that thin blood and improve muscle tone in the walls of blood vessels to enhance blood flow, especially to the brain.

4. Ginkgo helps to improve focus in the ADHD brain by inhibiting norepinephrine reuptake.

In a 2015 study, children and adolescents with ADHD received methylphenidate (20-30 mg/day) plus ginkgo Biloba (80-120 mg/day) or placebo for six weeks.

A 2000 double-blind, placebo-controlled study looked at the effects of standardized extract of ginkgo Biloba and standardized extract of Panax ginseng on various aspects of cognitive function in 256 healthy middle-aged volunteers.

Volunteers were asked to perform tests of attention and memory before their morning dosing on study days (weeks 0, 4, 8, 12, and 14). They performed the same tasks again at 1, 3, and 6 hours after their morning dose. The volunteers also completed questionnaires about mood states, quality of life, and sleep quality.

The ginkgo/ginseng combination was found significantly to improve memory quality. This effect represented an average improvement of 7.5% and reflected improvements to several different aspects of memory, including working and long-term memory. This enhancement to memory was seen throughout the 12-week dosing period and continued after a 2-week washout.

How Much Ginkgo Biloba Should I Take for ADHD?

Extracts of Ginkgo leaves contain flavonoid glycosides and terpenoids (ginkgolides, bilobalides). Ginkgo leaf extract may be taken at 80-160ml twice a day.

Studies have shown that ginkgo Biloba is best used together with ginseng to get better results in mental clarity. There is evidence that ginkgo leaf extract used in combination with American ginseng showed improvement in ADHD symptoms such as anxiety, hyperactivity, and impulsivity in children age 3 to 17-year-old.

The herb is generally well tolerated. Due to multiple case reports of bleeding, it should be used cautiously in patients on anticoagulant therapy and those with known blood clotting disorders, or before surgical or dental procedures.

Ginkgo biloba may interact with certain medications as well. Please consult your physician before starting a ginkgo Biloba extract supplement if you are taking any prescription medication for diabetes, blood pressure, seizure, etc.

Asian ginseng may overstimulate younger children. If this happens to your child, switch to American ginseng.

7. L-Theanine

Matcha green tea is more than just a drink. People have relied on the stress-relieving, sleep-promoting powers of matcha green tea for centuries.

Centuries ago, Japanese Zen monks first discovered that drinking matcha before long hours of meditation helped with their focus and kept them awake during long sessions of mental focus. Soon the Samurai adopted drinking matcha as a ritual to optimize their physical and cognitive performance during training and battle.

The secret is matcha's high concentration of the amino acid L-theanine, which reduces stress, and promotes a sense of peaceful focus.

Made from the entire leaf, matcha green tea's health benefits far outweigh those of traditional loose-leaf green tea.

L-Theanine is a non-protein amino acid found naturally in the green tea plant (Camellia sinensis) and in small amounts in Bay Bolete mushrooms. It is a precursor to GABA (gamma-aminobutyric acid) and supports healthy relaxation without drowsiness. Because it can cross the blood-brain barrier, L-theanine helps increase brain dopamine levels and helps support a healthy immune system.

One of the appealing aspects of L-theanine is that it works to relax without sedating. That can make L-theanine a good choice for people looking to enhance their "wakeful relaxation" without worrying about becoming sleepy and fatigued during the day.

3 Benefits of L-theanine for ADHD

1. Enhancing Attention, Focus, Memory, and Learning.

L-theanine, caffeine, and their combination seem to improve sustained attention and overall cognitive performance in children with **ADHD**.

Research shows L-theanine can increase attention span and reaction time in people who are prone to anxiety. It may help improve accuracy—one study shows that taking L-theanine reduced the number of errors made in a test of attention.

2. Reducing stress and anxiety.

L-theanine is an anxiolytic, which means it can reduce anxiety. Some anxiolytics, such as valerian and hops, have sedative effects. L-theanine, on the other hand, promotes relaxation and stress reduction without making you sleepy.

L-theanine has positive effects on both the mental and physical symptoms of stress, including lowering heart rate and blood pressure.

3. Improving sleep quality.

L-theanine may help people fall asleep more quickly and easily at bedtime, thanks to the relaxation boost it delivers. Research also shows L-theanine can improve the quality of sleep—not by acting as a sedative, but by lowering anxiety and promoting relaxation.

There's evidence that L-theanine may improve sleep quality in children with attention deficit hyperactivity disorder (ADHD). A study examined the effects of L-theanine on the sleep of boys ages 8-12. The study found that L theanine supplement worked safely and effectively to improve sleep quality, helping them sleep more soundly.

How Does L-Theanine Work for ADHD?

L-theanine raises levels of brain chemicals, such as GABA, serotonin, and dopamine, which regulate emotions, mood, concentration, alertness, sleep, appetite, energy, and other cognitive skills. Increasing levels of these calming brain chemicals promote relaxation and can help with sleep.

L-theanine also reduces levels of chemicals in the brain that are linked to stress and anxiety. It helps lower the stress hormone levels, such as corticosterone, and "excitatory" brain chemicals, such as glutamate.

When under stress, the body increases the production of certain hormones, including cortisol and corticosterone. These hormone changes inhibit some brain activity, including memory formation and spatial learning.

L theanine enhances alpha brain waves, which are associated with a state of "wakeful relaxation." That's the state of mind you experience when meditating, being creative "in the zone," or letting your mind wander in daydreaming.

Alpha waves are also present during REM sleep. L-theanine appears to trigger the release of alpha-waves, which enhances relaxation, focus, and creativity.

The following doses are based on amounts that have been investigated in scientific studies. It is recommended that users begin with the smallest suggested dose and gradually increase until it has an effect. For sleep, stress, and other uses: 100 mg to 400 mg.

Studies show that combining L-theanine and caffeine can improve attention span, enhance the ability to process visual information, and increase accuracy when switching from one task to another.

In combination with caffeine: 12-100 mg L-theanine, 30-100 mg caffeine.

Is L-theanine safe for Kids with ADHD?

L-theanine at relatively high doses was well tolerated in healthy adults with no significant adverse events.

One particular study concludes that 400mg L-theanine daily is safe and effective in improving some aspects of sleep quality in 8-12 years old boys diagnosed with ADHD.

8. Rhodiola Rosea

Using rhodiola rosea for mental focus with ADHD is not new. It's an herb with a long history in traditional medicine, and it is one of the most extensively studied herbs. If you have not heard of rhodiola, maybe you've heard of its other common names – *Arctic root or golden root or Siberian ginseng*. It is actually a very popular herb used in Europe and Russia.

Rhodiola is not a stimulant. It's an *adaptogenic herb, just like ginseng*. As an adaptogen, it helps the body resists stress both physically and emotionally while maintaining normal biological functions.

Rhodiola is used to reduce stress, combat fatigue, increase mental performance, and improve physical and mental fitness and resilience. In China and Russia, this herb is used to counter fatigue and help athletes recover from extreme physical activities.

Rosavins and salidrosides, the two main categories of compounds in rhodiola rosea, are responsible for the adaptogenic effects that regulate the stress hormone production, cortisol.

In milder ADHD cases, rhodiola *rosea* has been used as a solo treatment. It can be mentally stimulating while also emotionally calming. When used in conjunction with stimulants, rhodiola *rosea* is generally well tolerated.

3. Benefits of Rhodiola for ADHD

1. Rhodiola has been shown to improve concentration, focus and memory, and reducing symptoms of fatigue. In vitro studies of rhodiola rosea extract suggest that rhodiola rosea stimulates the reticular activating system and raise the levels of brain-calming chemicals, such as dopamine and serotonin. Serotonin is the neurotransmitter that makes you feel calm and happy. And dopamine is the one usually depleted in the prefrontal cortex of children with ADHD.

2. Rhodiola also helps with moderate depression and generalized anxiety. The active compounds, *Rasavins* and *salidrosides* are responsible for the antidepressant and anxiety-calming effects. Rosavins and salidrosides also stimulate epinephrine and norepinephrine production. These hormones promote a feeling of happiness and a sense of well-being.

3. Rhodiola rosea protects brain cells against oxidative injury; helps balance the stress-response system by preventing the excessive release of stress hormones like cortisol

HOW IS RHODIOLA TAKEN?

Physician supervision is advised when using rhodiola *rosea* as a sole or complementary treatment for ADHD. Be sure to let your physician know you plan to take rhodiola as it may interact with some of your prescription medication as it does influence the monoamine oxidase. This is especially true if you take any MAO inhibitors.

Rhodiola is most useful for junior high, high school, and college students who have to complete long papers and spend hours reading. It can be too stimulating for young children and is occasionally beneficial in children ages eight to 12.

For children 8–12 years old, very small doses can help improve symptoms of ADHD, particularly in cases in which increases in prescription stimulant doses are problematic.

The suggested dose for children is 50mg and 100-200mg for adults a day.

For children 12–18 years old, *rhodiola rosea* can be started at 50mg/day and increased by 50mg every 5–7 days, up to a maximum of 500mg/day and as long as it is well tolerated.

Rhodiola rosea should be given in the morning on an empty stomach to maintain its effect throughout the day.

Doses above 600mg per day are not recommended as these dosages have not yet been adequately studied, nor have they proven clinically useful.

Rhodiola is usually taken in capsule form. When purchasing rhodiola you are looking for two active ingredients – Rosavin (3%) and Salidroside (1%) ratio. Most formulas come in 3% rosavin and 1% salidroside.

Always start on a small amount and slowly increase to a dose that is controlling your symptoms and comfortable with you, even if it means you are not at the recommended dosage.

Just like ginseng, rhodiola should not be taken for a prolonged period as it may lose its effect with prolonged use. Take a break every 1-2 months.

SCIENTIFIC REFERENCES

"Science is organized knowledge…" Herbert Spencer

Acker WW, Plasek JM, Blumenthal KG, Lai KH, Topaz M, Seger DL, Goss FR, Slight SP, Bates DW, Zhou L. Prevalence of food allergies and intolerances documented in electronic health records. J Allergy Clin Immunol. 2017 Dec;140(6):1587-1591.e1. doi: 10.1016/j.jaci.2017.04.006. Epub 2017 May 31. PMID: 28577971; PMCID: PMC7059078.

American Psychiatric Association. (2013). Diagnostic and statistical manual of mental disorders (5th ed.). Washington, DC.

Altfas, Jules R. (September 2002). Prevalence of Attention Deficit/Hyperactivity Disorder Among Adults in Obesity Treatment. BMC Psychiatry. Vol. 29. doi:10.1186/1471-244X-2-9.

Altun H, Şahin N, Belge Kurutaş E, Güngör O. Homocysteine, Pyridoxine, Folate and Vitamin B12 Levels in Children with Attention Deficit Hyperactivity Disorder. Psychiatr Danub. 2018 Sep;30(3):310-316.

Amirmansour Alavi, Naeinia Forough, Fasihia Mostafa, Najafib Mohammad Reza Ghazvinic, Akbar Hasanzadehd. The effects of vitamin D supplementation on ADHD (Attention Deficit Hyperactivity Disorder) in 6–13 year-old students: A randomized, double-blind, placebo-controlled study. European Journal of Integrative Medicine. Volume 25, January 2019, Pages 28-33

Arwert, Lucia I., Jan Berend Deijen, and Madeleine L. Drent. "Effects of an oral mixture containing glycine, glutamine and niacin on memory, GH and IGF-I secretion in middle-aged and elderly subjects." Nutritional neuroscience 6.5 (2003): 269-275.

Bala KA, Doğan M, Kaba S, Mutluer T, Aslan O, Doğan SZ. Hormone disorder and vitamin deficiency in attention deficit hyperactivity disorder (ADHD) and autism spectrum disorders (ASDs). *J Pediatr Endocrinol Metab*. 2016;29(9):1077-1082. doi:10.1515/jpem-2015-0473

Barbaresi WJ, Colligan RC, Weaver AL, Voigt RG, Killian JM, Katusic SK. Mortality, ADHD, and psychosocial adversity in adults with childhood ADHD: a prospective study. Pediatrics. 2013 Apr;131(4):637-44. doi: 10.1542/peds.2012-2354. Epub 2013 Mar 4. PMID: 23460687; PMCID: PMC3821174.

Barkley RA, Fischer M, Smallish L, Fletcher K. Young adult outcome of hyperactive children: adaptive functioning in major life activities. J Am Acad Child Adolesc Psychiatry. 2006 Feb;45(2):192-202. doi: 10.1097/01.chi.0000189134.97436.e2. PMID: 16429090.

Barkley RA, Fischer M, Edelbrock CS, Smallish L. The adolescent outcome of hyperactive children diagnosed by research criteria: I. An 8-year prospective follow-up study. J Am Acad Child Adolesc Psychiatry. 1990 Jul;29(4):546-57. doi: 10.1097/00004583-199007000-00007. PMID: 2387789.

Barkley, R. A., & Fischer, M. (2019). Hyperactive Child Syndrome and Estimated Life Expectancy at Young Adult Follow-Up: The Role of ADHD Persistence and Other Potential Predictors. Journal of Attention Disorders, 23(9), 907–923. https://doi.org/10.1177/1087054718816164.

Biederman, Joseph et al.(2008). New Insights Into the Comorbidity Between ADHD and Major Depression in Adolescent and Young Adult Females. Journal of the American Academy of Child & Adolescent Psychiatry. Volume 47, Issue 4, 426 – 434. DOI: 10.1097/CHI.0b013e31816429d3.

Bilici M, Yildirim F, Kandil S, Bekaroğlu M, Yildirmiş S, Değer O, Ulgen M, Yildiran A, Aksu H. Double-blind, placebo-controlled study of zinc sulfate in the treatment of attention deficit hyperactivity disorder. Prog Neuropsychopharmacol Biol Psychiatry. 2004 Jan;28(1):181-90.

Benoit Chassaing, Manish Kumar, Mark T. Baker, Vishal Singh, and Matam Vijay- Kumar. Mammalian Gut Immunity. Biomed J. 2014 ; 37(5): 246–258. doi:10.4103/2319-4170.130922.

Bos DJ, Oranje B, Veerhoek ES, Van Diepen RM, Weusten JM, Demmelmair H, Koletzko B, de Sain-van der Velden MG, Eilander A, Hoeksma M, Durston S. 2015. Reduced Symptoms of Inattention after Dietary Omega-3 Fatty Acid Supplementation in Boys with and without Attention Deficit/Hyperactivity Disorder. Neuropsychopharmacology. 2015. 40(10):2298-306

Bourre JM. Effects of nutrients (in food) on the structure and function of the nervous system: update on dietary requirements for brain. Part 1: micronutrients. J Nutr Health Aging. 2006 Sep-Oct;10(5):377-85.

Checa-Ros A, Haro-García A, Seiquer I, Molina-Carballo A, Uberos-Fernández J, Muñoz-Hoyos A. Early monitoring of fatty acid profile in children with attention deficit and/or hyperactivity disorder under treatment with omega-3 polyunsaturated fatty acids. Minerva Pediatr. 2018 Nov 7.

Chou WJ, Lee MF, Hou ML, Hsiao LS, Lee MJ, Chou MC, Wang LJ. Dietary and nutrient status of children with attention-deficit/hyperactivity disorder: a case-control study. Asia Pac J Clin Nutr. 2018;27(6):1325-1331.

Chung W, Jiang S, Paksarian D, et al. Trends in the Prevalence and Incidence of Attention-Deficit/Hyperactivity Disorder Among Adults and Children of Different Racial and Ethnic Groups. JAMA Netw Open. 2019;2(11):e1914344. doi:https://doi.org/10.1001/jamanetworkopen.2019.14344

Curry AE, Metzger KB, Pfeiffer MR, Elliott MR, Winston FK, Power TJ. Motor Vehicle Crash Risk Among Adolescents and Young Adults With Attention-Deficit/Hyperactivity Disorder. *JAMA Pediatr.* 2017;171(8):756–763. doi:10.1001/jamapediatrics.2017.0910

Davis NO1, Kollins SH. Treatment for co-occurring attention deficit/hyperactivity disorder and autism spectrum disorder. Neurotherapeutics. 2012 Jul;9(3):518-30. doi: 10.1007/s13311-012-0126-9

Dehbokri N, Noorazar G, Ghaffari A, Mehdizadeh G, Sarbakhsh P, Ghaffary S. Effect of vitamin D treatment in children with attention-deficit hyperactivity disorder. *World J Pediatr.* 2019;15(1):78-84. doi:10.1007/s12519-018-0209-8

Den Heijer AE, Groen Y, Tucha L, Fuermaier AB, Koerts J, Lange KW, Thome J, Tucha O. Sweat it out? The effects of physical exercise on cognition and behavior in children and adults with ADHD: a systematic literature review. J Neural Transm (Vienna). 2017 Feb;124(Suppl 1):3-26.

Dolina S, Margalit D, Malitsky S, Rabinkov A. Attention-deficit hyperactivity disorder (ADHD) as a pyridoxine-dependent condition: urinary diagnostic biomarkers. *Med Hypotheses.* 2014;82(1):111-116. doi:10.1016/j.mehy.2013.11.018

DuPaul, G. J., Weyandt, L. L., O'Dell, S. M., & Varejao, M. (2009). College Students With ADHD: Current Status and Future Directions. Journal of Attention Disorders. 13(3), 234–250. https://doi.org/10.1177/1087054709340650.

Durá-Travé T, Gallinas-Victoriano F. Caloric and nutrient intake in children with attention deficit hyperactivity disorder treated with extended-release methylphenidate: analysis of a cross-sectional nutrition survey. JRSM Open. 2014 Feb 3;5(2):2042533313517690.

Durá Travé T, Diez Bayona V, Yoldi Petri ME, Aguilera Albesa S. [Dietary patterns in patients with attention deficit hyperactivity disorder]. An Pediatr (Barc). 2014 Apr;80(4):206-13.

Ek, U., Westerlund, J., Holmberg, K., Fernell, E. (July 2008). Self-Esteem in Children with Attention and/or Learning Deficits: The Importance of Gender. Acta Pædiatrica. 97: 1125-1130. doi:10.1111/j.1651-2227.2008.00894.x.

Elia, J., Ambrosini, P., & Berrettini, W. (2008). ADHD characteristics: I. Concurrent co-morbidity patterns in children & adolescents. Child and adolescent psychiatry and mental health, 2(1), 15. doi:10.1186/1753-2000-2-15.

Elshorbagy HH, Barseem NF, Abdelghani WE, et al. Impact of Vitamin D Supplementation on Attention-Deficit Hyperactivity Disorder in Children. *Ann Pharmacother.* 2018;52(7):623-631. doi:10.1177/1060028018759471

Esparham A, Evans RG, Wagner LE, Drisko JA. Pediatric Integrative Medicine Approaches to Attention Deficit Hyperactivity Disorder (ADHD). Children (Basel). 2014 Aug 27;1(2):186-207.

Evans S, Ling M, Hill B, Rinehart N, Austin D, Sciberras E. Systematic review of meditation-based interventions for children with ADHD. Eur Child Adolesc Psychiatry. 2018 Jan;27(1):9-27.

Fanjiang G, Kleinman RE. Nutrition and performance in children. Curr Opin Clin Nutr Metab Care. 2007 May;10(3):342-7.

Faraone SV., Spencer TJ., Montano CB., Biederman J. (2004). Attention-Deficit/Hyperactivity Disorder in Adults: A Survey of Current Practice in Psychiatry and Primary Care. Arch Intern Med.164(11):1221–1226. doi:10.1001/archinte.164.11.1221.

Farida El Baza, Heba Ahmed Al Shahawi, Sally Zahra, Rana Ahmed, Abdel Hakim_Magnesium supplementation in children with attention deficit hyperactivity disorder. Egyptian Journal of Medical Human Genetics. Volume 17, Issue 1, January 2016, Pages 63-70

Farr SA, Price TO, Banks WA, Ercal N, Morley JE. Effect of alpha-lipoic acid on memory, oxidation, and lifespan in SAMP8 mice. *J Alzheimers Dis*. 2012;32(2):447-455. doi:10.3233/JAD-2012-120130

FDA Drug Safety Communication: Safety Review Update of Medications used to treat Attention-Deficit/Hyperactivity Disorder (ADHD) in children and young adults. Assessed at https://www.fda.gov/drugs/drug-safety-and-availability/fda-drug-safety-communication-safety-review-update-medications-used-treat-attention

Galler JR, Ramsey F, Solimano G. The influence of early malnutrition on subsequent behavioral development III. Learning disabilities as a sequel to malnutrition. Pediatr Res. 1984 Apr;18(4):309-13. doi: 10.1203/00006450-198404000-00001. PMID: 6718088.

Galler JR, Ramsey F, Solimano G, Lowelled WE. The Influence of Early Malnutrition on Subsequent Behavioral Development: II. Classroom Behavior. Journal of the American Academy of Child Psychiatry Volume 22, Issue 1, January 1983, Pages 16-22

Gokcen C, Kocak N, Pekgor A. Methylenetetrahydrofolate reductase gene polymorphisms in children with attention deficit hyperactivity disorder. *Int J Med Sci*. 2011;8(7):523-528. doi:10.7150/ijms.8.523

Hae-Jin Ko, Inbo Kim, Jong-Bae Kim, Yong Moon, Min-Cheol Whang, Keun-Mi Lee, and Seung-Pil Jung.Journal of Child and Adolescent Psychopharmacology. Nov 2014.501-508.

Hager, Klaus, et al. "Alpha-lipoic acid as a new treatment option for Alzheimer type dementia." *Archives of gerontology and geriatrics* 32.3 (2001): 275-282.

Hinz M, Stein A, Neff R, Weinberg R, Uncini T. Treatment of attention deficit hyperactivity disorder with monoamine amino acid precursors and organic cation transporter assay interpretation. *Neuropsychiatr Dis Treat*. 2011;7:31-38. Published 2011 Jan 26. doi:10.2147/NDT.S16270

Hoogman M, Bralten J, Hibar DP, Mennes M, Zwiers MP, Schweren LSJ, et al. Subcortical brain volume differences in participants with attention deficit hyperactivity disorder in children and adults: a cross-sectional mega-analysis. VOLUME 4, ISSUE 4, P310-319, APRIL 01, 2017

Hurt, E.A., Arnold, L.E. & Lofthouse, N. Dietary and Nutritional Treatments for Attention-Deficit/Hyperactivity Disorder: Current Research Support and Recommendations for Practitioners. *Curr Psychiatry Rep* **13,** 323 (2011). https://doi.org/10.1007/s11920-011-0217-z

Jing Gan, Peter Galer, Dan Ma, Chao Chen, and Tao Xiong.Journal of Child and Adolescent Psychopharmacology.Nov 2019.670-687.http://doi.org/10.1089/cap.2019.0059

Kennedy DO. B Vitamins and the Brain: Mechanisms, Dose and Efficacy--A Review. *Nutrients*. 2016;8(2):68. Published 2016 Jan 27. doi:10.3390/nu8020068

Kessler, R. C., Adler, L., Barkley, R., Biederman, J., Conners, C. K., Demler, O., Zaslavsky, A. M. (2006). The Prevalence and Correlates of Adult ADHD in the United States: Results from the National Comorbidity Survey Replication. American Journal of Psychiatry. 163, 716-723. doi:10.1176/appi.ajp.163.4.716.

Konofal, Eric & Lecendreux, Michel & Deron, Juliette & Marchand, Martine & Cortese, Samuele & Zaïm, Mohammed & Mouren, Marie & Arnulf, Isabelle. (2008). Effects of Iron Supplementation on Attention Deficit Hyperactivity Disorder in Children. Pediatric neurology. 38. 20-6. 10.1016/j.pediatrneurol.2007.08.014.

Kozielec T. Assessment of magnesium levels in children with attention deficit hyperactivity disorder. Magnes Res, 10 (2) (1997), pp. 143-148

Kozielec T, Starobrat-Hermelin B. Assessment of magnesium levels in children with attention deficit hyperactivity disorder (ADHD). Magnes Res. 1997 Jun;10(2):143-8.

Lange KW, Hauser J, Lange KM, Makulska-Gertruda E, Nakamura Y, Reissmann A, Sakaue Y, Takano T, Takeuchi Y. The Role of Nutritional Supplements in the Treatment of ADHD: What the Evidence Says. Curr Psychiatry Rep. 2017 Feb;19(2):8.

Larson, K., Russ, S. A., Kahn, R. S., & Halfon, N. (2011). Patterns of comorbidity, functioning, and service use for US children with ADHD, 2007. Pediatrics, 127(3), 462–470. doi:10.1542/peds.2010-0165.

Lee SH, Park WS, Lim MH. Clinical effects of korean red ginseng on attention deficit hyperactivity disorder in children: an observational study. *J Ginseng Res*. 2011;35(2):226-234. doi:10.5142/jgr.2011.35.2.226

Lee, Steve S et al. (2011). Prospective Association of Chilhood Attention-Deficit/Hyperactivity Disorder (ADHD) and Substance Use and Abuse/Dependence: A Meta-Analytic Review. Clinical Psychology Review. Vol. 31,3: 328-41. doi:10.1016/j.cpr.2011.01.006.

Lopez-Corcuera, Beatriz, Arjan Geerlings, and Carmen Aragon. "Glycine neurotransmitter transporters: an update." Molecular membrane biology 18.1 (2001): 13-20.

López-Vicente, Mónica et al. (June 2019). Prenatal Omega-6: Omega-3 Ratio and Attention Deficit and Hyperactivity Disorder Symptoms. The Journal of Pediatrics. Volume 209, 204 – 211.e4. DOI: https://doi.org/10.1016/j.jpeds.2019.02.022.

Lynskey MT, Fergusson DM.. Childhood conduct problems, attention deficit behaviors, and adolescent alcohol, tobacco, and illicit drug use. J Abnorm Child Psychol. 1995;23:281–302.

Lyon MR, Cline JC, Totosy de Zepetnek J, Shan JJ, Pang P, Benishin C. Effect of the herbal extract combination Panax quinquefolium and Ginkgo biloba on attention-deficit hyperactivity disorder: a pilot study. *J Psychiatry Neurosci*. 2001;26(3):221-228.

Merkel RL Jr, Nichols JQ, Fellers JC, Hidalgo P, Martinez LA, Putziger I, Burket RC, Cox DJ. Comparison of On-Road Driving Between Young Adults With and Without ADHD. J Atten Disord. 2016 Mar;20(3):260-9. doi: 10.1177/1087054712473832. Epub 2013 Feb 11. PMID: 23400213.

M. Mousain-Bosc, M. Roche, A. Polge, D. Pradal-Prat, J. Rapin, J.P. Bali. Improvement of neurobehavioral disorders in children supplemented with magnesium-vitamin B6. I. Attention deficit hyperactivity disorders
Mag Res, 19 (1) (2006), pp. 46-52

M. Mousain-Bosc, M. Roche, J. Rapin, J.P. Bali. Magnesium VitB6 intake reduces central nervous system hyperexcitability in children
J Am Col Nutr, 23 (5) (2004), pp. 545S-548S

Markel, C., Wiener, J. (2014). Attribution Processes in Parent-Adolescent Conflict in Families of Adolescents With and Without ADHD. Canadian Journal of Behavioural Science/Revue Canadienne Des Sciences Du Comportement. 46, 40-48. doi:10.1037/a0029854.

Magdy M. Mahmoud, Abdel-Azeem M. El-Mazary, Reham M. Maher, Manal M. Saber. Zinc, ferritin, magnesium and copper in a group of Egyptian children with attention deficit hyperactivity disorder. Ital J Pediatr, 37 (2011), pp. 60-67

Matthews RT, Yang L, Browne S, Baik M, Beal MF. Coenzyme Q10 administration increases brain mitochondrial concentrations and exerts neuroprotective effects. *Proc Natl Acad Sci U S A*. 1998;95(15):8892-8897. doi:10.1073/pnas.95.15.8892

Mousain-Bosc M, Roche M, Polge A, Pradal-Prat D, Rapin J, Bali JP. Improvement of neurobehavioral disorders in children supplemented with magnesium-vitamin B6. I. Attention deficit hyperactivity disorders. *Magnes Res*. 2006;19(1):46-52.

Melissa L. Danielson, Rebecca H. Bitsko, Reem M. Ghandour, Joseph R. Holbrook, Michael D. Kogan & Stephen J. Blumberg. (Jan. 24, 2018). Prevalence of Parent-Reported ADHD Diagnosis and Associated Treatment Among U.S. Children and Adolescents, 2016. Journal of Clinical Child & Adolescent Psychology, 47:2, 199-212, DOI: 10.1080/15374416.2017.1417860.

Mian, A., Jansen, P., Nguyen, A., et. al. (April 2019). Children's Attention-Deficit/Hyperactivity Disorder Symptoms Predict Lower Diet Quality but Not Vice Versa: Results from Bidirectional Analyses in a Population-Based Cohort. The Journal of Nutrition. Volume 149, Issue 4. Pages 642–648. https://doi.org/10.1093/jn/nxy273.

Michael H. Bloch, M.D., M.S.a, Omega-3 Fatty Acid Supplementation for the Treatment of Children With Attention-Deficit/Hyperactivity Disorder Symptomatology: Systematic Review and Meta-Analysis. Journal of the American Academy of Child & Adolescent Psychiatry, Volume 50, Issue 10, 991 - 1000

Milte CM, Parletta N, Buckley JD, Coates AM, Young RM, Howe PR. Increased Erythrocyte Eicosapentaenoic Acid and Docosahexaenoic Acid Are Associated With Improved Attention and Behavior in Children With ADHD in a Randomized Controlled Three-Way Crossover Trial. J Atten Disord. 2015 Nov;19(11):954-64.

Molz, Patrícia and Nadja Schröder. "Potential Therapeutic Effects of Lipoic Acid on Memory Deficits Related to Aging and Neurodegeneration" *Frontiers in pharmacology* vol. 8 849. 12 Dec. 2017, doi:10.3389/fphar.2017.00849

Ng QX, Ho CYX, Chan HW, Yong BZJ, Yeo WS. Managing childhood and adolescent attention-deficit/hyperactivity disorder (ADHD) with exercise: A systematic review. Complement Ther Med. 2017 Oct;34:123-128.

Norman LJ, Carlisi C, Lukito S, Hart H, Mataix-Cols D, Radua J, Rubia K. Structural and Functional Brain Abnormalities in Attention-Deficit/Hyperactivity Disorder and Obsessive-Compulsive Disorder: A Comparative Meta-analysis. JAMA Psychiatry. 2016 Aug 1;73(8):815-825.

Packer, Lester, and Enrique Cadenas. "Lipoic Acid: Energy Metabolism and Redox Regulation of Transcription and Cell Signaling." *Journal of Clinical Biochemistry and Nutrition* 48, no. 1 (2010): 26–32. doi:10.3164/jcbn.11-005FR.

Parletta N, Niyonsenga T, Duff J. Omega-3 and Omega-6 Polyunsaturated Fatty Acid Levels and Correlations with Symptoms in Children with Attention Deficit Hyperactivity Disorder, Autistic Spectrum Disorder and Typically Developing Controls. PLoS One. 2016 May 27;11(5):e0156432.

Paul, Steven. "GABA and Glycine". American College of Neuropsychopharmacology. Accessed at https://acnp.org/g4/GN401000008/Default.htm

Pellow J, Solomon EM, Barnard CN. Complementary and alternative medical therapies for children with attention-deficit/hyperactivity disorder (ADHD). Altern Med Rev. 2011 Dec;16(4):323-37.

Percinel I, Yazici KU, Ustundag B. Iron Deficiency Parameters in Children and Adolescents with Attention-Deficit/Hyperactivity Disorder. Child Psychiatry Hum Dev. 2016 Apr;47(2):259-69.

Pelsser LM, Frankena K, Toorman J, Savelkoul HF, Dubois AE, Pereira RR, et al. Effects of a restricted elimination diet on the behaviour of children with attention-deficit hyperactivity disorder (INCA study): a randomised controlled trial. The Lancet. VOLUME 377, ISSUE 9764, P494-503, FEBRUARY 05, 2011

Quinn, P. O. (2005). Treating Adolescent Girls and Women with ADHD: Gender–Specific Issues. Journal of Clinical Psychology. 61: 579-587. doi:10.1002/jclp.20121.

Richardson AJ, Burton JR, Sewell RP, Spreckelsen TF, Montgomery P (2012) Docosahexaenoic Acid for Reading, Cognition and Behavior in Children Aged 7–9 Years: A Randomized, Controlled Trial (The DOLAB Study). PLOS ONE 7(9): e43909. Assessed at https://doi.org/10.1371/journal.pone.0043909

Richardson AJ, Puri BK. A randomized double-blind, placebo-controlled study of the effects of supplementation with highly unsaturated fatty acids on ADHD-related symptoms in children with specific learning difficulties. Prog Neuropsychopharmacol Biol Psychiatry. 2002 Feb;26(2):233-9.

Reinblatt, Shauna P., et al. (April 2015). Pediatric Loss of Control Eating Syndrome: Association with Attention–Deficit/Hyperactivity Disorder and Impulsivity. Int. J. Eat. Disord., 48: 580-588.

Roberts JR, Dawley EH, Reigart JR. Children's low-level pesticide exposure and associations with autism and ADHD: a review. Pediatr Res. 2018 Oct 8.

Roberts JR, Karr CJ; Council On Environmental Health. Pesticide exposure in children. Pediatrics. 2012 Dec;130(6):e1765-88.

Rucklidge, J. et al. (2001). Psychiatric, Psychosocial, and Cognitive Functioning of Female Adolescents With ADHD. Journal of the American Academy of Child & Adolescent Psychiatry. Volume 40, Issue 5, 530 – 540. doi: 10.1097/00004583-200105000-00012.

Sawni A Attention-deficit/hyperactivity disorder and complementary/alternative medicine. Adolesc Med State Art Rev. 2008 Aug;19(2):313-26, xi.

Shrier LA, Harris SK, and Kurland M. et al. Substance use problems and associated psychiatric symptoms among adolescents in primary care. Pediatrics. 2003 111:e699–e705.

Simon, V., Czobor, P., Bálint, S., Mészáros, Á, & Bitter, I. (2009). Prevalence and Correlates of Adult Attention-Deficit Hyperactivity Disorder: Meta-Analysis. British Journal of Psychiatry. 194(3), 204-211. doi:10.1192/bjp.bp.107.048827.

S J, Arumugam N, Parasher RK. Effect of physical exercises on attention, motor skill and physical fitness in children with attention deficit hyperactivity disorder: a systematic review. Atten Defic Hyperact Disord. 2018 Sep 27.

Smalley, Susan L. et al. Familial Clustering of Symptoms and Disruptive Behaviors in Multiplex Families With Attention-Deficit/Hyperactivity Disorder. (September 2000). Journal of the American Academy of Child & Adolescent Psychiatry. Volume 39, Issue 9, 1135 – 1143. https://doi.org/10.1097/00004583-200009000-00013.

Stacey Ageranioti Bélanger, Michel Vanasse, Schohraya Spahis, Marie-Pierre Sylvestre, Sarah Lippé, François l'Heureux, Parviz Ghadirian, Catherine-Marie Vanasse, and Emile Levy. Omega-3 fatty acid treatment of children with attention-deficit hyperactivity disorder: A randomized, double-blind, placebo-controlled study. Paediatr Child Health. 2009 Feb; 14(2): 89–98. doi: 10.1093/pch/14.2.89

Tseng PT Cheng YS, Yen CF, Chen YW, Stubbs B, Whiteley P, Carvalho AF, Li DJ, Chen TY, Yang WC, Tang CH, Chu CS, Yang WC, Liang HY, Wu CK, Lin PY. Peripheral iron levels in children with attention-deficit hyperactivity disorder: a systematic review and meta-analysis. Sci Rep. 2018 Jan 15;8(1):788.

Uçkardeş Y, Tekçiçek M, Ozmert EN, Yurdakök K. The effect of systemic zinc supplementation on oral health in low socioeconomic level children. Turk J Pediatr. 2009 Sep-Oct;51(5):424-8. Assessed at https://www.ncbi.nlm.nih.gov/pubmed/20112596

Upadhyaya HP, Rose K, and Wang W. et al. Attention-deficit/hyperactivity disorder, medication treatment, and substance use patterns among adolescents and young adults. J Child Adolesc Psychopharmacol. 2005 15:799–809.

van Emmerik-van Oortmerssen, K., van de Glind, G., van den Brink, W., Smit, F., Crunelle, C. L., Swets, M., Schoevers, R. A. (April 2012). Prevalence of Attention-Deficit Hyperactivity Disorder in Substance Use Disorder Patients: A Meta-Analysis and Meta-Regression Analysis. Drug and Alcohol Dependence. Volume 122, Issues 1–2. Pages 11-19. doi:10.1016/j.drugalcdep.2011.12.007.

Verlaet AAJ, Maasakkers CM, Hermans N, Savelkoul HFJ. Rationale for Dietary Antioxidant Treatment of ADHD. Nutrients. 2018 Mar 24;10(4). pii: E405.

Visser, S. N. et al. Trends in the Parent-Report of Health Care Provider-Diagnosed and Medicated Attention-Deficit/Hyperactivity Disorder: United States, 2003–2011. Journal of the American Academy of Child & Adolescent Psychiatry,Volume 53, Issue 1, 34 – 46.e2. DOI: 10.1016/j.jaac.2013.09.001.

Vohr BR, Poggi Davis E, Wanke CA, Krebs NF. Neurodevelopment: The Impact of Nutrition and Inflammation During Preconception and Pregnancy in Low-Resource Settings. Pediatrics. 2017 Apr;139(Suppl 1):S38-S49.

Walkup, John T. et al. (January 2014). Beyond Rising Rates: Personalized Medicine and Public Health Approaches to the Diagnosis and Treatment of Attention-Deficit/Hyperactivity Disorder. Journal of the American Academy of Child & Adolescent Psychiatry. Volume 53, Issue 1, 14 – 16. DOI: https://doi.org/10.1016/j.jaac.2013.10.008.

Widenhorn-Müller K, Schwanda S, Scholz E, Spitzer M, Bode H. Effect of supplementation with long-chain ω-3 polyunsaturated fatty acids on behavior and cognition in children with attention deficit/hyperactivity disorder (ADHD): a randomized placebo-controlled intervention trial. Prostaglandins Leukot Essent Fatty Acids. 2014 Jul-Aug;91(1-2):49-60.

Wood, Amber. "Glycine or Collagen?" AmberWood Health. October 17, 2018. https://amberwoodhealth.ca/glycine-or-collagen/

Yamadera, K.; Chiba, S.; Bannai, M.; Takahashi, M., Nakayama, K., Glycine ingestion improves subjective sleep quality in human volunteers, correlating with polysomnographic changes, Sleep and Biological Rhythms 5 (2007).

Yektaş Ç, Alpay M, Tufan AE. Comparison of serum B12, folate and homocysteine concentrations in children with autism spectrum disorder or attention deficit hyperactivity disorder and healthy controls. *Neuropsychiatr Dis Treat*. 2019;15:2213-2219. Published 2019 Aug 6. doi:10.2147/NDT.S212361
Yvonne Kelly, John Kelly and Amanda Sacker. Changes in Bedtime Schedules and Behavioral Difficulties in 7 Year Old Children. Pediatrics November 2013, 132 (5) e1184-e1193.

Zhang J, Díaz-Román A, Cortese S Meditation-based therapies for attention-deficit/hyperactivity disorder in children, adolescents and adults: a systematic review and meta-analysis. Evid Based Ment Health. 2018 Aug;21(3):87-94.

Photo credits go to original owners, whoever you are. Most pictures are free stock photos from Adobe Spark, Pixabay and Canva.

To all original owners of pictures and memes borrowed in this book, I appreciate your artistic ability in creating such beautiful pictures to be enjoyed with everyone.

MEDICAL DISCLAIMER

This book offers health, fitness and nutritional information and is designed for educational purposes only. You should not rely on this information as a substitute for, nor does it replace, professional medical advice, diagnosis, or treatment. If you have any concerns or questions about your health, you should always consult with a physician or other health-care professional. Do not disregard, avoid or delay obtaining medical or health related advice from your health-care professional because of something you may have read on this site. The use of any information provided on this site is solely at your own risk.

Developments in medical research may impact the health, fitness and nutritional advice that appears here. No assurance can be given that the advice contained in this site will always include the most recent findings or developments with respect to the particular material.

You should consult your physician or other health care professional before starting this or any other fitness program to determine if it is right for your needs. This is particularly true if you (or your family) have a history of high blood pressure or heart disease, or if you have ever experienced chest pain when exercising or have experienced chest pain in the past month when not engaged in physical activity, smoke, have high cholesterol, are obese, or have a bone or joint problem that could be made worse by a change in physical activity. Do not start this fitness program if your physician or health care provider advises against it. If you experience faintness, dizziness, pain or shortness of breath at any time while exercising you should stop immediately.

If you are in the United States and think you are having a medical or health emergency, call your health care professional, or 911, immediately.

Made in United States
North Haven, CT
10 April 2024